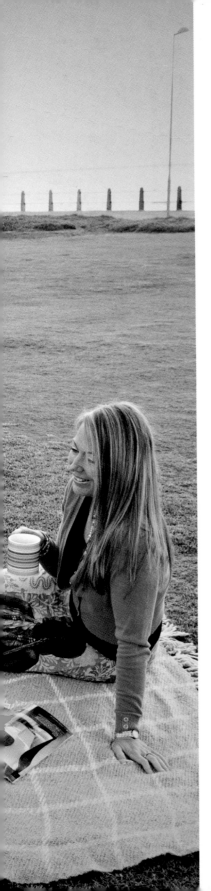

KU-478-178

LOW-CARB LIVING
for Families

Monique le Roux Forslund

Photography by Mikael Eriksson,
Monica Dart and Monique le Roux Forslund

Acknowledgements

I would like to thank the three hearts in my life: my children – Daniel, Amilia and Lisa – who taste, eat and enjoy my food. I truly appreciate your opinions and constant support. You are the best!

A huge thank you to my mom, who has taught me to experiment in the kitchen with new tastes and ideas, and to believe in myself. And to my dad, who knows all about how and what to barbecue.

Thank you also to my colleagues at Cosmos Montessori pre-school for your patience with my ideas and suggestions, and for sharing an interest in providing good and healthy food for children at our school.

Finally, thank you to all the children who have passed through Cosmos's doors. You have shown me how the right food makes for satisfied children. You have been my inspiration.

Published in 2013 by Struik Lifestyle
an imprint of Penguin Random House South Africa (Pty) Ltd
Company Reg. No. 1953/000441/07
The Estuaries, 4 Oxbow Crescent, Century Avenue, Century City 7441
PO Box 1144, Cape Town, 8000

www.randomstruik.co.za

Adapted from *LCHF fö* [hela familjen], published by Pagina Förlags AB Optimal Förlag in 2012

Copyright © in published edition: Penguin Random House South Africa (Pty) Ltd 2013
Copyright © in text: Monique le Roux Forslund 2013
Copyright © in photographs: Pagina Förlags AB/Optimal Förlag 2013

All rights reserved. No [part of this publication may be reproduced], stored in a retrieval system or transmitted, in any f[orm or by any means], electronic, mechanical, [photocopying, recording or otherwise, without [the written permission of the publishers] and copyright holders.

LONDON BOROUGH OF WANDSWORTH		
9030 00005 1665 1		
Askews & Holts	04-Aug-2016	
613.2833	£14.99	
	WW16008701	

Publisher: Linda de Villiers
Managing editor: Cecilia Barfield
Editor and indexer: Joy Clack (Bushbaby Editorial Services)
Designer: Helen Henn
Photographers: Mikael Eriksson, Monica Dart, M Industries and Monique le Roux Forslund
Proofreader: Laetitia Sullivan (Bushbaby Editorial Services)

Reproduction by Hirt & Carter Cape (Pty) Ltd
Printing and binding: 1010 Printing International Ltd, China

ISBN: 978-1-43230-124-8 (Print)
ISBN: 978-1-43230-314-3 (ePub)
ISBN: 978-1-43230-315-0 (PDF)

DISCLAIMER:
The opinion and information in this book are those of the author and cannot replace the advice of a qualified health professional for an individual's specific health requirements. The author and publishers assume no liability for any consequences or inconvenience sustained by any person using this book or the information given in it.

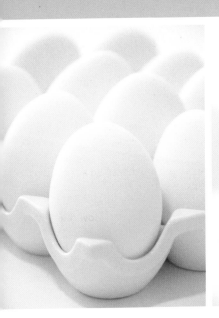 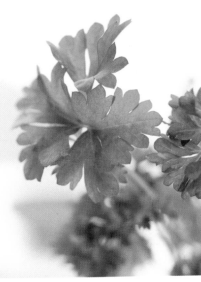 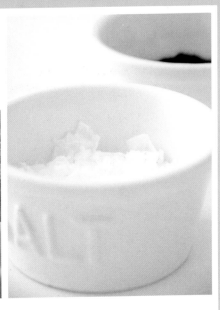

Contents

Forewords

In 1977 a vegan, Nick Mottern, with no formal training in the nutritional sciences irrevocably changed the future of nutritional choices around the globe. On the invitation of the United States Senate Select Committee on Nutrition and under the chairmanship of Senator George McGovern, Mr Mottern set about drafting new eating guidelines for all Americans; guidelines which would become the global standard. His finished masterpiece, the *1977 Dietary Goals for the United States*, would become the defining landmark in the modern history of nutrition. So influential are those guidelines that one can now consider two eras of nutrition – the periods before and after the *1977 Dietary Goals*.

Despite an absence of irrefutable scientific backing, the *1977 Dietary Goals* recommended that from that time forth, all healthy humans must ingest only those high-carbohydrate diets that include 7–12 servings of cereals and grains a day with little fat and a complete absence of 'unhealthy' fats. That humans had eaten diets rich in fat and protein and without cereals and grains for all but the last 2–12 000 years of their 3.5 million-year march to becoming *Homo sapiens* was forgotten.

Industry was not slow to grasp the implications of this exciting new business opportunity. Very soon it learned that foods with the low fat content required by Mr Mottern's *Dietary Goals* tasted little better than cardboard. And so to increase the palatability they added first sugar – later high fructose corn syrup – and then salt in increasing amounts, transforming foods from their traditional function as sources of nutrition to vehicles of addiction. For they had discovered that foods with just the right amounts of fat, sugar and salt produce the 'bliss' moment – the irresistible urge to eat and keep eating that blissful product regardless of the excess calories ingested and the inevitable unhealthy consequences. And then in their final triumph, they marketed these addictive, unnatural, man-engineered products as healthy because they were 'low fat'. It was a masterstroke matched only by the achievements of the tobacco industry a generation before.

There was no evidence then, nor is there any now, that this low-fat, high-carbohydrate diet would improve the health of the world. Instead, what transpired was entirely predictable on the basis of what has been known since 1825 – humans fed an excess of carbohydrates become fat, just as do farm animals eating the same foods. So the past 30 years has witnessed a medical tsunami of obesity and diabetes overwhelming the entire globe as processed foods specifically designed for their addictive properties have progressively ousted natural foods from our diets.

Surprisingly, no one is prepared to take responsibility for this disaster, even though the writings of Michael Moss now reveal that the food industry has been aware – since 1997 – that their addictive foods are the cause of the global obesity/diabetes epidemic. Nor is anyone ready to explain how this epidemic might be reversed – even though the evidence of how this can be achieved is clear. Instead, the targeted victims of this epidemic are told that they are too lazy and gluttonous. If only they would eat less and to exercise more, their obesity and diabetes would disappear. But this, too, is wrong. In fact, there is a far easier solution.

As two previously corpulent individuals who were supposedly lazy and gluttonous, the author of this book, Monique le Roux Forslund, and I beg to differ. We discovered, as do all who try, that the more intensively we worked at regulating our body weights with exercise and diet, the larger we grew. We learned that our corpulence had almost nothing to do with how much exercise we did. Instead, the more we exercised and the less fat we ate, the hungrier we became. And so, eating according to Mr Mottern's *Dietary Goals,* we just grew fatter and more disheartened.

Then, by different routes, we both discovered the solution to our common problem. We found out that we both suffer from carbohydrate intolerance, also known medically as insulin resistance. When those of us who are insulin resistant ingest Mr Mottern's 'healthy' high-carbohydrate diet, we are unable to store more than a marginal amount of carbohydrates in the normal body stores – our liver and muscles. Instead, we secrete too much of the fat-building hormone insulin, which converts the excess carbohydrates into fat. This, in turn, induces a chain of secondary reactions leading to obesity and ultimately diabetes, heart disease and certain cancers, as well as an accelerated mental and physical decline with ageing.

So it turns out that for us, like all humans who suffer from the same condition, Mr Mottern's dietary solution is the cause and not the cure of our anguish. Dietary fat, the very food that his *Dietary Goals* have demonised, is the single most important component of the diet that will make us healthy.

Monique le Roux Forslund, born in Cape Town, has been living in Sweden since 1992. Long before I had learned this critical dietary lesson, Monique had not only discovered this truth but had set about educating the compatriots of her adopted country about the importance of eating a diet high in fat and low in carbohydrates – the LCHF eating plan. Through a popular website and a cookbook in Swedish she became instrumental in helping to convert Swedes to LCHF. Today up to 25% of 9 million Swedes now follow this LCHF eating plan.

Now those South Africans who wish to become healthier by following the LCHF can also benefit from Monique's passion. For in these pages is the first South African cookbook devoted exclusively to LCHF recipes. It is a local version of her highly successful Swedish original. This book fills a need that is being felt ever more urgently in this country as health-conscious South Africans wishing to experience the benefits of the LCHF eating plan begin to consider their dietary options. Here, for the first time, they will discover the recipes they seek, presented in an attractive and accessible manner. The publication of this book represents a key milestone in the progress of South Africans towards healthier eating choices. May your health benefit as much from its wisdom as have Monique and I.

Professor Tim Noakes OMS, MBChB, MD, DSc, PhD (hc)

Discovery Health Professor of Exercise and Sports Science
University of Cape Town and Sports Science Institute of South Africa

Literature:

Moss, Michael. *Salt, Sugar, Fat. How the Food Giants Hooked Us*. Random House, New York, 2013.
Taubes, Gary. *Good Calories, Bad Calories*. Anchor Books, New York, 2007.

This book has the potential to implode the myth that low-fat diets are good for you. The topic of low-carb high-fat eating for children is very controversial, but how can you dispute the benefits of eating natural foods, such as fish, meat, vegetables, berries, nuts and butter, that make you feel full; that are homemade using good and basic ingredients, without unnecessary additives?

What has happened to the world? When did it become the norm to feed children artificial light products instead of real and natural foods?

Health authorities around the world still recommend low-fat products to children. It's advice based on the fear of natural fats which took off during the eighties, at about the same time as obesity increased drastically, in both adults and children.

However, a growing number of doctors and researchers today realise that the fear of fat was a mistake. Replacing natural fat with bad carbohydrates like sugar and white flour is not a good idea. Your cholesterol profile will not improve because you avoid eating fat, and it has now been proven that there are no fewer cases of heart disease in people eating artificial low-fat margarine.

Low-fat and diet products do not make you feel as full as full-fat products. This can, ironically, cause you to eat more and gain weight. And the same thing happens to your children. Feeling hungry also makes it difficult for them to concentrate in school, leading older children to buy energy drinks and candy during their school breaks and causing younger children to nag their parents for snacks.

Monique le Roux Forslund – health coach, mother of three and Montessori teacher – has vast experience with children. In this book she gives advice on better alternatives available for children and families to eat. Nourishing food that makes you feel full; food that will satisfy your children and help them focus and concentrate in school.

This book is not about cutting out all carbs or feeding children a strict low-carb high-fat diet. Healthy children with normal weight can still eat root vegetables and fruits, and all children will benefit from less exposure – at least at home – to the worst parts of westernised junk food: sugar, flour and hard-to-pronounce additives.

My 18-month-old daughter is already on the waiting list for Monique's pre-school, where I know the children are fed good and nourishing food. I truly hope that the fear of fat will be long gone by the time my daughter starts school and I hope that she, and all other children, will always eat good food and never feel the need to stay hungry.

Read this book. Then spread the knowledge so that common sense will prevail and so that our children will get the good start in life that they deserve.

Andreas Eenfeldt MD

Specialist in family medicine

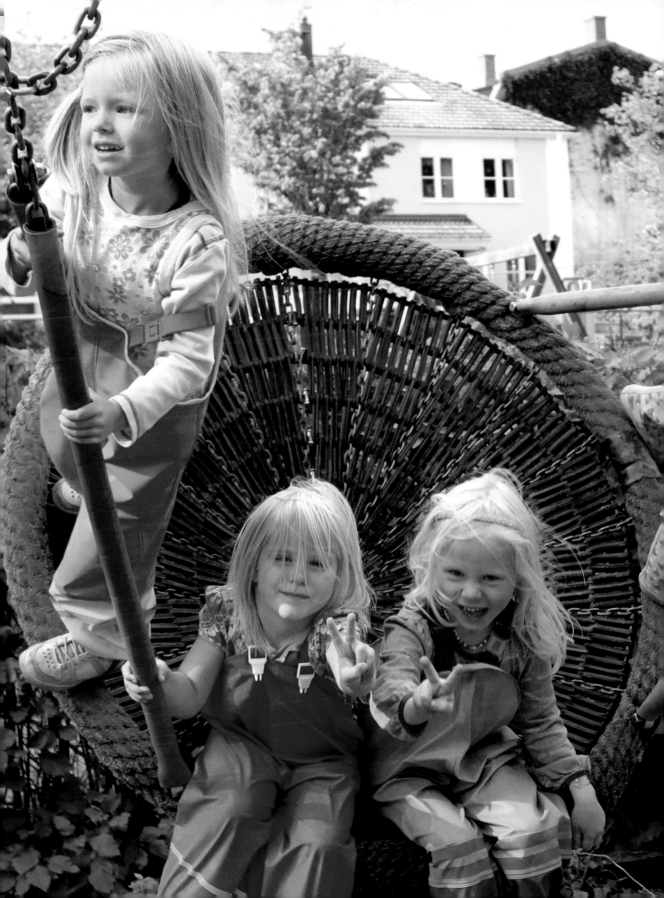

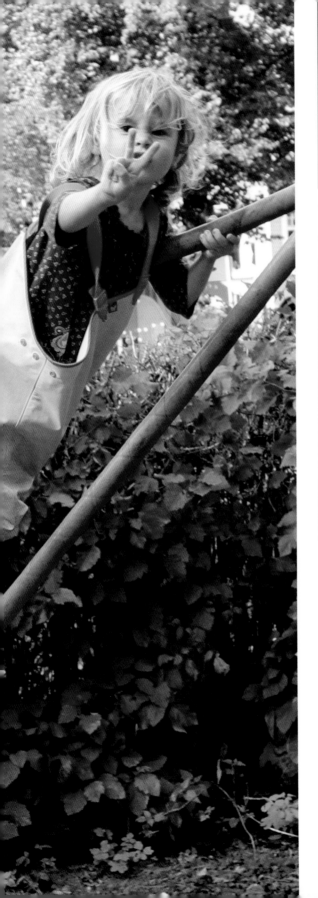

Introduction

Our children are the future. Let's help provide them with a healthy lifestyle.

The most important thing to think about is good, basic food of the best quality and nutrition available. My aim is to avoid as many additives, flavourings and colorants as possible. Children should eat natural, healthy foods that fill them up and help them stay full while at the same time providing the right amount of energy.

As a health coach, teacher, mom of three and with over 20 years of experience working with children, I would like to share my experiences and knowledge with you on the effects food has on children's health.

Over the years I have seen how food not only affects the individual child but also groups of children. I have observed how children react to fast-working carbohydrates, how they 'turbo energise' and how sugar affects them in a negative way. Concentration ability decreases due to bad food choices.

My hope is to provide you with easy-to-follow, practical tips on good food for growing children. Food that helps children to concentrate and to sit still in class. Food that provides the right amount of positive energy and food that makes them full and satisfied for hours.

Natural food with high nutritional value is the basis of our children's health.

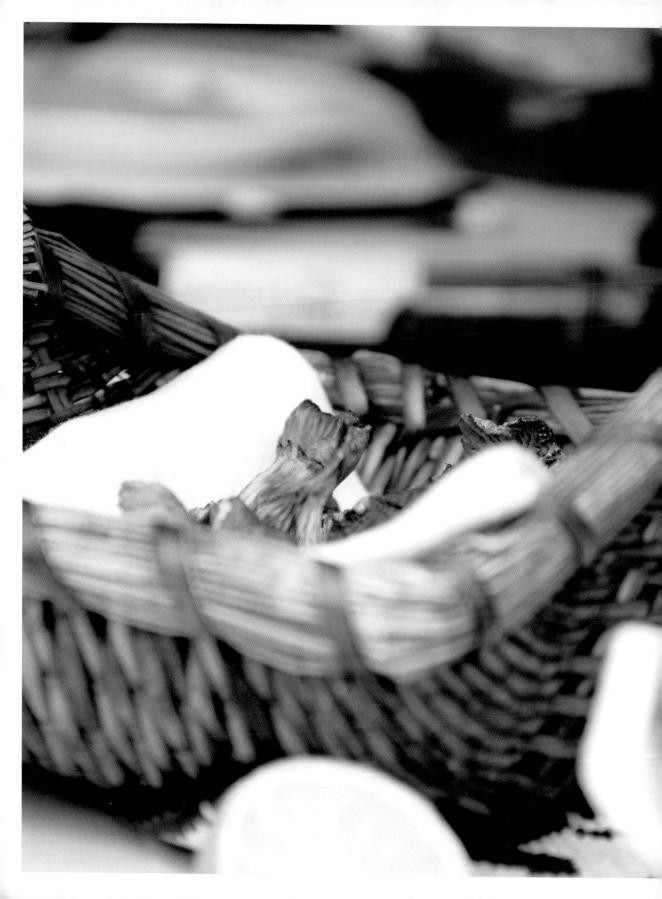

Natural food and healthy fats

I use the definition LCHF (low carb high fat). This way of eating, or lifestyle, is about decreasing carbohydrates and increasing consumption of natural fats. This is beneficial for all of us, not only for children. In doing this you will feel fuller and satisfied for a longer period of time, avoid blood sugar peaks and diminish cravings and the need to eat sweet things or constantly snack.

If you eat meat, fish, eggs, fat, nuts, berries and vegetables you will provide the body with all the nutrients it needs: vitamins, minerals and antioxidants.

Carbohydrates

Carbohydrates (carbs) consist of sugar, fibre and starch. Sugar is easily distinguishable due to its sweet taste. Starch, however, can be more difficult to discern. Starch is found in foods such as flour, bread, oats, cereals, porridge, pasta, potatoes, rice, corn, brown rice and bulgur. Carbs are also found in milk, yoghurt, vegetables, cereals, nuts, cakes, biscuits, popcorn, chips, beans, sweets and candy, soda and rice cakes.

Carbs are quickly broken down into glucose (blood sugar) and therefore raise your blood sugar. High blood sugar stimulates insulin production in the pancreas and the insulin in turn opens up the cells in the body to take in the blood sugar and turn it into energy. A high amount of insulin turns blood sugar into fat and increases body fat storage. Too much insulin stops the burning of fat and can lead to an unhealthy body.

When you decrease the amount of carbohydrates you consume, you don't need to be afraid of eating fats or calories, as they will not store as fat in your body. Avoid choosing foods that are high in fat and high in sugar (carbs).

Parts of the brain need glucose to function properly. Carbohydrates turn to glucose in the liver, but this is not the only way of producing glucose for the brain. The liver can also produce glucose from proteins. This process is called gluconeogenesis.

We are all individuals and are therefore more or less tolerant of different foods and amounts of carbohydrates. The effect of eating something sweet or something that raises blood sugar can vary from one person to another. This is why I mention how sensitive the body can be to food. For those who are sensitive to carbohydrates, a portion of fruit or a helping of potatoes can be sufficient to trigger cravings for the wrong foods and/or something sweet to eat. Children, too, tolerate different amounts of carbohydrates for the same reason.

Carbohydrates are what I call turbo energy. If a child has the choice, he or she will most likely choose carbohydrates before other foods, and especially carbs that are extremely high in sugar, such as white bread and white pasta instead of wholewheat foods. They tend to choose food that provides them with the most energy, which may also give them a 'kick'.

Consuming more carbohydrates than the body can tolerate will result in too much sugar in the bloodstream. Initially it feels like a boost of energy, but shortly afterwards the blood sugar levels decrease, along with the ability to concentrate. This leads to the need to eat again in order to gain more energy, which will quickly diminish again and will leave you feeling tired and listless. It's a relentless cycle.

Bearing this in mind, imagine how this can affect a child, or children in general, on a daily basis. A breakfast in the form of cereal, fruit yoghurt, bread, juice or maybe flavoured milk is a breakfast with total turbo energy. The children then go off to school where they perhaps have a snack in the form of a biscuit, fruit or sandwich. More turbo energy. And then along comes lunch time and the turbo energy intake continues with whatever high-carb food they eat, such as sandwiches, hotdogs, pasta or rice with a meal. During this time the child is expected to listen, concentrate, sit still and absorb what the teacher is saying. Some children can cope, but many cannot. They have too much turbo energy in their bodies. Sitting still can be difficult enough, never mind concentrating at the same time.

It is important that children consume good fat in their diet, and here I emphasise the importance of using real butter and not margarine. The fat in their diet is what makes them feel satisfied and keeps them full for longer. A lack of fat will cause children to become hungry again shortly after eating a meal or snack, and at the same time make them inattentive.

Your child and LCHF

Imagine children eating a nourishing and filling breakfast that is low in carbs and high in fat. This will keep them full for a long period of time and help them be more focused. A low-carb and high-fat breakfast consists of, for example, eggs, tea, low-carb bread or low-carb crisp bread with a generous amount of butter and a filling topping such as salami, ham, cheese, avocado or egg with mayonnaise.

After such a breakfast children are able to concentrate better, sit still and listen for a longer period of time. They are also calmer, have a calm tummy and feel full and satisfied all morning until lunch time. If they eat a nourishing and filling lunch that contains proteins, fats and minimal carbs, this will provide them with the right amount of energy to play after lunch and then go in and work again, without having any difficulty focusing or having cravings or hunger pangs for something more to eat. With less excess turbo energy I will go so far as to say, from my experience working with children, that even conflicts will diminish.

I encourage every parent to try this LCHF lifestyle for themselves and their children. Observe how your children react and how sensitive they are to carbs. I think most parents will be pleasantly surprised at the improvement in their children's health and wellbeing.

Fat

Fat is good for you, fat is nourishing and we all need to consume it. Fat is what makes us feel full and satisfied. Fat is also necessary in order for our bodies to absorb important fat-soluble vitamins, such as vitamin A, D, E and K, and is important for our immune system. Eating fat also increases the rate at which your body burns fat.

Your choice of fat, however, is important. You should choose good fats, natural fats and fats that humans have been eating since the very beginning and that are found naturally in our diet.

Fats that are good to eat are:
- Saturated fat in meat, minced meat, chicken skin, full-fat or heavy cream, cheese, butter and extra virgin coconut oil, preferably organic.
- Monounsaturated fat found in avocados, olives and nuts.
- Polyunsaturated fat found in fatty fish such as mackerel and salmon. Omega-3 from fatty fish is a polyunsaturated fat that is vital to our wellbeing.

The fats you need to avoid in your diet are all trans fats, interesterified fat, hydrogenated fats and partially hydrogenated fats. Margarine in all forms should be avoided, as it is artificial fat that has been bleached, coloured and flavoured with artificial flavouring to make it as similar as possible to real butter. Margarine has a long shelf life, does not become rancid and is cheap, but it is not good for the body.

Children and adults should eat full-fat and natural foods. All diet and light products should be avoided because the manufacturer has reduced or removed the healthy fats and most likely replaced them with carbohydrates, for example flavoured yoghurts.

Always use full-fat (full-cream) products: milk, crème fraîche, cream, yoghurt, cheese, mayonnaise, etc. These high in fat products make you feel full and satisfied and are more natural. The wonderful thing about fat is that it has no impact on blood sugar levels or insulin.

Protein

Proteins are the building blocks of the body. They consist of vital amino acids, which are largely responsible for the production of our muscles, nails and hair. In other words, everyone needs to eat proteins.

In adults, there are eight different amino acids that the body cannot create by itself. Children need 10 different amino acids. Eggs, meat, fish and fowl are foods that are high in protein. An egg has a protein composition that is good for your body and contains everything that the body needs, except vitamin C. If there is one product that is worth spending that little bit extra on in order to get a higher quality product, it is organic eggs.

Low carb for families

Choosing low-carb food with good fat content is, in general, normal and natural food. By eating low-carb food your blood sugar levels will remain constant and will not put strain on your insulin system. Staying satisfied for a longer period of time will prevent cravings for something sweet.

A low-carb diet can also help to drastically reduce health problems such as gastric problems, heartburn, skin problems, acne, depression, sleep disorders, mood swings, joint pains, lifeless hair, migraines, irregular blood sugar curves, diabetes, eating disorders, fibromyalgia, PMS, obesity, asthma and sugar addiction. A LCHF diet will provide the body with all the nourishment it needs, and you can eat your way to good health.

This book is not about cutting out all carbs or about feeding children a strict low-carb diet. It is about finding your way through the jungle of products and information in our society, leading to a life of natural foods and products that satisfy hunger, banish cravings and provide a healthy lifestyle.

My goal is to give tips and inspiration for a healthy way of living with good alternatives for the whole family. This includes a small amount of carbohydrates in fruits, berries and vegetables for children and teenagers. Adults can choose a stricter version of the low-carb way of eating to meet personal needs and goals. Observe how much your body tolerates and how sensitive you and your children are to various carbohydrates.

Eat, live and enjoy!

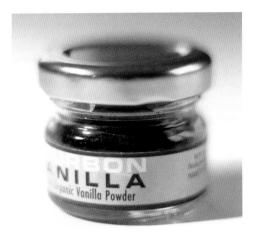

Conversions

Metric	US cups
5 ml	1 tsp
15 ml	1 Tbsp
60 ml	4 Tbsp or ¼ cup
80 ml	⅓ cup
125 ml	½ cup
160 ml	⅔ cup
200 ml	¾ cup
250 ml	1 cup

Oven temperatures

Celsius (°C)	Fahrenheit (°F)	Gas mark
100 °C	200 °F	¼
110 °C	225 °F	¼
120 °C	250 °F	½
140 °C	275 °F	1
150 °C	300 °F	2
160 °C	325 °F	3
180 °C	350 °F	4
190 °C	375 °F	5
200 °C	400 °F	6
220 °C	425 °F	7
230 °C	450 °F	8
240 °C	475 °F	9

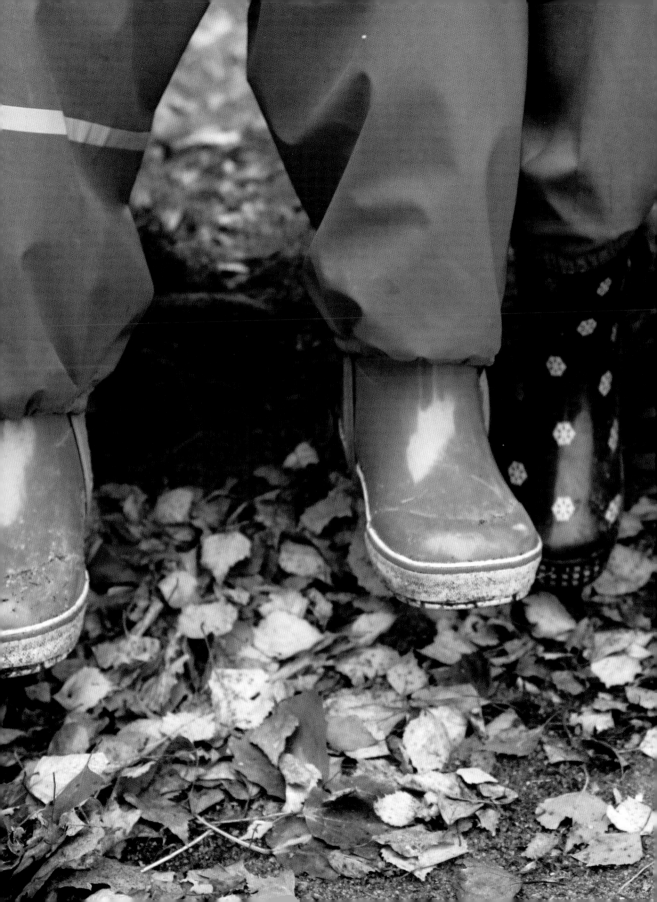

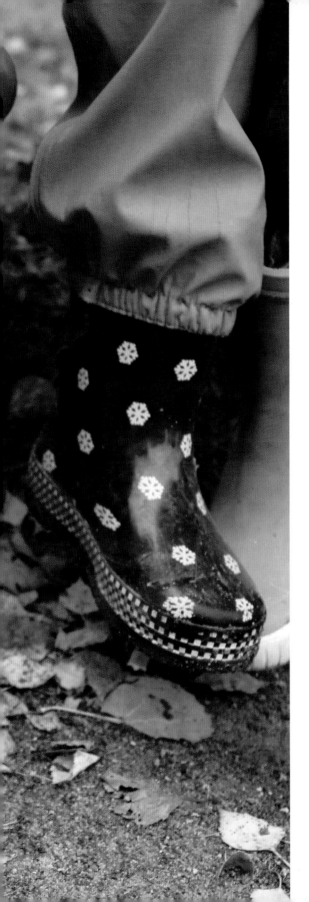

Practical low carb for families

A family consists of several individuals with several opinions and several different tastes. As we age, our knowledge, habits and tastes change. A small child will most often eat what is being served, but teenagers often choose what they want to eat.

Accept that there are different opinions in all families, especially when it comes to food, and that prohibiting certain food items can be difficult. Try to be flexible while sticking to the guidelines within the low-carb diet. Listen to your children and try to meet them halfway. I do, however, prohibit one thing at home, and that is MSG/E621/ yeast extract/glutamate (many names for the same thing). Monosodium glutamate (MSG) is a common food additive used to enhance the flavour of certain foods. Extensive studies have been done on MSG and many believe that it has very negative effects on the body.

My goal is to emphasise the importance of nourishing and healthy foods for the whole family. The ideas, recipes and tips included in this book are to help inspire you to prepare good food that is both energy rich and nourishing. There are also ideas for healthy fast foods for those who are pressed for time.

Making it work for your family

You need to answer the following questions to be able to establish the extent of the lifestyle changes you wish to make. Work together to see what you can accomplish as a family.

- Does everyone in the family want to change their way of eating, or is it only the adults who wish to do so?
- Should you prepare different meals to suit the family or should the person making the food decide what is going to be served?
- Should sodas, juice and biscuits or cakes be allowed as soon as friends come over to visit or are there any other alternatives that can be served instead?
- Do desserts have to be sweet?
- Do we need something sweet after dinner?
- Do we need to eat anything after dinner?

Food to have at home

Below is a list of good food alternatives to stock up on at home. This way you and the kids will be able to find something healthy to prepare whenever necessary.

Dairy products
Butter
Brie cheese and/or other soft cheeses
Full-fat fresh cream
Full-fat milk
Greek or Bulgarian yoghurt
Crème fraîche
Full-fat cheese (Cheddar, Gouda, etc.)
Feta cheese
Full-fat mayonnaise

Proteins
Eggs (preferably organic)
Chicken
Salami (good quality)
Ham, smoked beef or pastrami
Fish
Meat (beef, lamb, pork, venison)
Minced meat
Mackerel (tinned is good to have at home)
Tuna (in water; avoid sunflower oil)

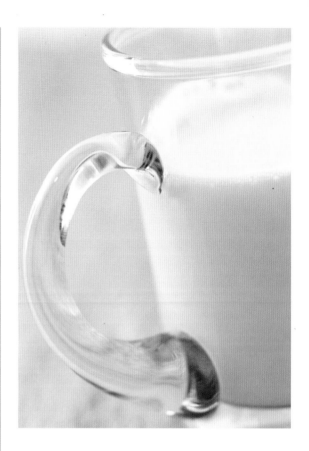

Vegetables
There are vitamins and antioxidants in vegetables. There are also carbohydrates, but this is where the 'low' comes into low carb. Whenever possible, choose vegetables that grow above the ground. For some, root vegetables (from below the ground) can also work, but only if you do not have weight issues or diabetes. All vegetables are fine for children, but limit potatoes as much as possible.
Avocado
Asparagus
Lettuce, rocket, fresh spinach and other dark, leafy greens
Leek
Tomato
Cabbage
Broccoli
Cauliflower
Brussels sprouts
Aubergine (egg plant, brinjal)

Baby marrow (courgette, zucchini)
Mushroom
Onion
Squash
Peppers
Olives

Dressings
Extra virgin olive oil
Spices and herbs
Vinegar (avoid balsamic vinegar where possible)

Fruit
If your body can handle fruit (not recommended during weight loss or for diabetics), eat it together with a meal or at least with some source of protein.

Apple
Pear
Citrus fruits
Pomegranate
Berries

Fats
Organic coconut oil is the best oil to use for making food and it tolerates heat better than all other oils and increases your body's fat burning. A spoonful every morning is very good for you and it works well in both coffee and tea.

Ghee is also very good for making food. Do not fry food in olive oil as it becomes oxidised. When you heat oil, the oil's characteristics change. Some oils that are otherwise healthy become unhealthy when heated above certain temperatures.

Coconut oil
Butter
Mayonnaise
Nuts
Avocado
Olive oil

Nuts (always raw, unsalted)
Macadamia
Almonds
Brazil nuts
Walnuts
Hazelnuts

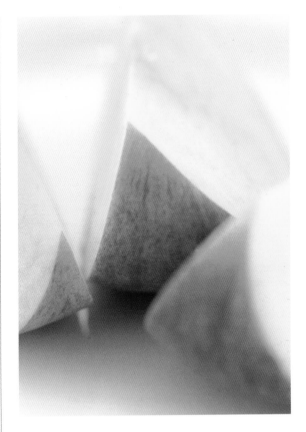

Liquids
Tap water
Sparkling water
Coffee
Tea (green, red, black)

What to avoid
Always read the label before buying food items – you will soon learn what various foods contain and what to look for, or which food items to avoid. In the beginning this does take some time, but you will quickly get into it and will be reading and understanding food labels without realising it.

The ingredients on food labels are listed in descending order, with the first ingredient making up most of the product. In other words, the first item is what the product contains most of. Soon you will learn what to avoid and which alternatives to choose instead. You will also understand which products are of better quality and are therefore more suitable to buy.

All diet, light and sugar-free products

These products are usually made from chemicals and sometimes also sugar. Many diet products or fat-free items are richer in carbohydrates as the manufacturers add more carbs when removing the fats.

Margarine

All kinds of margarines! If it says margarine on the container, don't buy it.

Sugar

If sugar is listed as an ingredient on a product label, especially if it's number one to three, the product should be avoided.

An easy rule to follow is that the amount of carbohydrates should not exceed 3–5 grams carbs per 100 gram serving. Even if the amount is within an acceptable range, this does not mean that the product is okay to eat in unlimited amounts.

Grains (and pulses)

All foods that contain flour. Grains and pulses in general are to be avoided.

Sweeteners

All products that contain sweeteners such as aspartame, sucralose, etc. In just about all products that are called 'sugar free' there are sweeteners instead of sugar.

Flavour enhancer

Monosodium glutamate (MSG) is also known as E621, glutamate and yeast extract. It is found in many spice blends, fast foods, ready-made or frozen meals, sausages, bacon, cookies, bread (some), gravy packets, bastings, and so on.

If there is MSG in a product it should be stated on the label. MSG is unhealthy and not good for your body (see page 15).

Snacks

Chips
Candy
Flavoured nuts
Soda
Juice
Ice cream

Other

Rice
Pasta
Shop-bought sauces, such as tomato sauce (ketchup), chilli sauce, sweetened mustard
Fruit yoghurt
Pudding
Rice cakes
Beans or peas or corn
Sweet fruits high in fructose, such as melons, grapes, mango, plums, nectarines and banana

Fussy eaters

Some children simply refuse to eat, or eat only small amounts and fiddle with the rest of the food on the plate. This can cause many parents to worry. Children don't have the same focus on food and eating as adults do because they are busy learning so many things in life and that occupies them instead. Children eat when they need to eat and usually eat better both before and after a new stage of development.

Make sure meal times are family times, where everyone sits around the same table. Adults are our children's role models and children will therefore imitate and do what they see and not what we say.

Encouraging children to eat

The aromas of food being prepared in the kitchen increases our appetite, and the same applies to children. The smell of your neighbour's barbecue or the aroma of freshly baked bread wafting from a nearby bakery can easily make you feel a bit hungry or feel cravings for something to eat.

Encourage your children to be a part of the food-making process and let them be involved in preparing various dishes, especially things they like. Trust them with a proper small knife and involve them in the chopping and slicing.

Avoid nagging, bribery and rewarding when it comes to meals and eating. Don't tell your children to eat up everything, but rather encourage them to taste all the items on the plate. Explain that food is good for them and they need to eat food in order to have enough energy to play and learn.

There are various reasons why a child may refuse to eat. One of them is if the child is tired and lacks energy.

In this case a small snack can be effective in improving the child's mood and appetite. A child who is rested eats better than a child who is very tired.

Bear in mind that many small meals and snacks during the day can also affect your child's eating habits at meal times. Many times children never get the opportunity to feel hungry as we as loving parents keep feeding them throughout the day. Find the balance that works for your family.

Accept that your children may want to feed themselves – 'I can' – and encourage them to do so. Allow the time it takes for your children to learn to eat on their own and ignore the mess that might be made. A spoon in each hand will encourage your child to eat using utensils instead of fingers. Not all children like being fed while others are happy to be fed for years. It is your responsibility as a parent to help them learn to do it themselves.

Try to have at least one thing on your child's plate that they recognise or like, especially if you are introducing something new to eat. If you know, for instance, that your child likes cheese, then include a few pieces of cheese on the plate when you are introducing a new dish or new foods.

Encourage your child to help set the table with nice napkins or some flowers so that meal times are positive. Participation is a part of eating.

Teenagers

The teenage years are about searching for independence. They can entail new friends, shopping for clothes, finding and discovering new activities, financial responsibility, going to parties and staying up much later in the evenings. Teenagers want to make their own choices and decisions.

Although diet and the way of eating will have an effect on a teenager, there are no easy or obvious solutions to increase awareness for healthy eating. Today's youth are surrounded by unhealthy fast foods, particularly via the media and advertisements. Fast food is easy to obtain and group peer pressure should also be taken into account when it comes to teenagers and their eating habits.

To encourage your teenager to eat a low-carb diet can work very well if he or she is receptive to the idea and generally interested in diet and health. If your teenager is not interested, the chances are low that he or she will change their way of eating because one of their parents wants them to.

But don't hesitate to talk about good food and good food choices every now and then, about what is good and what is less healthy. Providing knowledge in small doses without nagging or demands is important. The knowledge that your teenager gains during these years will hopefully stick with them throughout life, and one day it will become useful.

Bad habits and eating stages

With unlimited access to junk food, a teenager can easily get stuck in 'fast food mode'.

Many teenagers start their day by sleeping through or skipping breakfast. When they get to school, they often buy some kind of fast food from the school shop/ cafeteria and then perhaps buy lunch, which again consists of fast foods and/or diet and light products with minimal nourishment. They may also buy something on their way home from school as they feel they need something to give them an energy kick.

At home you as the parent are hopefully able to provide a healthy and filling meal, which is when your teenager has the first proper meal of the day.

Observe your teenager and his or her eating habits. Is there anything you can do to increase food awareness and to get them to eat healthier meals more often?

Eating stages are also very common amongst teenagers. This occurs most often during periods of growth when your teenager suddenly eats large amounts of food, all the time, all day long. They are constantly hungry. Help out by stocking up on good food that is easy for him or her to prepare, and that is also filling.

Teenagers and weight

Always avoid talking about dieting with your teenager. Being overweight is a very sensitive topic. Dieticians and many teachers at schools encourage more exercise and less food in order to lose weight, but you should explain to your teenager that it is about WHAT they eat and not the AMOUNT they are eating (calories) or exercising that may be causing weight issues (if there is a weight issue). Explain that he or she does not need to diet but instead needs to focus on what they are eating, and which choices are better than others.

Be a good example because you project various signals to your child. Don't complain about your own body, weight, size or other people's appearances.

Teenagers and exercise

Teenagers that are active and work out or train do tolerate more carbohydrates compared to those that sit still and play a lot of computer or TV games. Many professional athletes eat a low-carb diet and have shown very good training results.

Use my snack suggestions on pages 139–149 as foods to eat before and/or after a work-out. The egg milk (protein drink) on page 41 is great in combination with training. Don't eat less than 3 hours before a tough work-out and feel free to eat something directly after the work-out.

In my experience, protein shakes are quite popular amongst teenagers – part of peer pressure? Most protein shakes are sweetened, but there are some unsweetened protein shakes available if he or she really wants to drink protein shakes. Generally I think protein shakes are unnecessary as you can make your own healthier protein drink at home.

If your teenager has chosen to change to a low-carb lifestyle, it is advisable to ease off on training and working out for a couple of weeks to give the body time to adjust to fat adaptation as its energy source.

Healthy alternatives

Place emphasis on the importance of good food choices and how bad foods can have a negative effect on the body. Monosodium glutamate is one of the bad choices and when it comes to this I am a nagging mom. If there is one thing you want your child to understand and listen to, this could be it! Don't eat anything that contains MSG.

Encourage good and healthy products and real foods, and avoid all low-fat, sugar-free or other diet products. Natural foods include butter, cream, coconut oil and vegetables to mention a few. Encourage your teenager to eat high-quality vegetables, protein, eggs and fish. If you can get this far with your teenager, then you are winning the 'fast food battle'.

Most teenagers will likely still buy junk food, chips and candy, but even here there are better or worse choices to be made. Here are a few tips on some 'better than' foods:

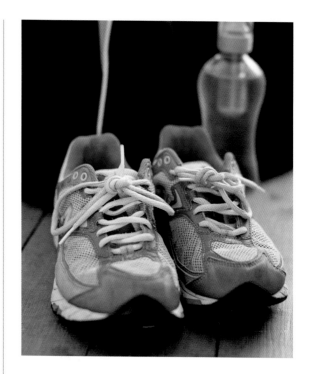

- Choose juice or soda instead of energy drinks.
- Choose sparkling flavoured water instead of juice or soda.
- Choose natural chips instead of flavoured chips.
- Choose salty peanuts instead of chips.
- Choose chocolate instead of candy (which contains chemicals and colorants).
- Choose a whole package of ham instead of jam on a sandwich.
- Choose homemade hot cocoa with cream instead of the instant chocolate powders available.
- Choose lots of sauce with food instead of lots of pasta.
- Choose more fat and carbohydrates instead of no fat and carbohydrates (the fat makes you feel full).

Availability

Make sure that there are good food choices at home, in the pantry and in the fridge and allow your teenager to decide how much he or she wants to eat. I often think I have a fridge full of food at home, yet my teenagers open the fridge door and say there is nothing to eat! Ask your teenager to write a shopping list of favourite foods and then you can choose the better things to buy from that list. And buy lots!

Buy a soda maker, soda or sparkling water to reduce the amount of sodas being bought. Many teenagers don't have the time or patience to make food from scratch so prepare some dishes in bulk and freeze them in portion sizes – these are easy to reheat and provide a ready meal.

I never buy pasta, cereals, rice, juice or soda and have a rule that if my teenagers wish to eat any of these items, they have to go and buy it themselves with their own money. This they do, at times. At home they eat the low-carb meals that I prepare, but outside of our home they eat as many other teenagers do. At least they have a lot of knowledge about what is good and what is not!

Fructose

Fructose is the sugar we most commonly find naturally in fruits and vegetables and is one of the sweetest sugars that exist. Normal white sugar consists of 50% glucose and 50% fructose. Modern research shows that a large amount of fructose is the worst carbohydrate for our health and weight. A hundred years ago the average amount of sugar consumed per person was 15 grams a day. Today this amount is five times more. Fructose increases body weight because it is the carbohydrate that the body most easily converts into fat. It also affects insulin in a negative way.

Fruit is a very 'sensitive' subject for many people when it comes to discussing healthy food alternatives. People can react very strongly when we talk about fruit and sugar in the same sentence and as something negative. The good thing about fruit is that it is very tasty. It's natural candy, I usually say. When it comes to nourishment, however, you will find much more in vegetables than in fruit. The ground where fruit trees are planted often lacks nourishment and the fruit we eat today is very different to how fruit was many years ago. Today the fruits are larger, sweeter and are often not grown naturally.

I think it's fine for children to eat fruit in reasonable amounts, and preferably together with a meal or protein such as cheese or eggs. This way it will have less effect on blood sugar levels.

Additives

Additives are added to food to preserve or to enhance flavour or taste. Pickling (with vinegar) and salting food has been used for centuries as a way of preserving foods, but more processed foods are being used today and many more additives have been introduced. Each additive has its own unique number, what we know as 'E numbers'.

Legislation dictates that all additives must be specified on food labels of all foods. The producer can choose whether to use the E number or to write the full name of the additives that are being used. I won't list all the E numbers but will mention a few that I would like to warn you about.

E numbers from E620 to E650 are taste enhancers. These are used in foods where the original product is of such poor quality or made from poor-quality ingredients that the taste has either vanished or deteriorated or where the product just tastes so bad that even spices cannot improve the taste. E621 is almost the same as yeast extract, which is another name for something that has a similar function as E621 (MSG). It is also known as a taste enhancer.

These taste enhancers may cause headaches, sweating, nausea, heartburn, dizziness and chest pains. MSG/E621 is banned in many children's foods – that should tell you quite a bit.

Aromas are also used in products of poorer quality so that the natural flavour or taste will be enhanced. Butter aroma, for instance, is very common, as is smoke aroma in bacon. I try not to buy any products with added aroma, which is an artificial aroma. It is always better to keep your choices as natural as possible.

Colorants are also additives to watch out for. They have the E numbers E100 to E180. These are cosmetic additives and are often used when a product loses its colour during the production process. Many producers add colorants to food products to make them look more appetising.

If you look at candy and how children are most likely to choose the most colourful candies from the selection on offer, then you can understand why producers use these colorants. Azo colorants/dyes can cause sensitivity reactions, such as rashes, asthma, runny noses and eyes. There are also suspicions about the effects of food dyes on hyperactivity.

Particular colorants/food dyes that you should watch out for are:

- E102 tartrazine (yellow)
- E104 quinoline yellow (yellow)
- E110 para (orange)
- E122 azorubine (red)
- E124 cochineal red (red)
- E129 allura red AC

Colorants/food dyes can be found in many products, including ham, margarine, marzipan, ready-made cakes, jam, curry, tinned berries, sausage, sauce, yoghurt, cereal, and candy and soda. My tip is to write a small note about which E numbers to avoid and keep that note in your wallet so that you can easily check when doing your shopping.

We know very little about the foods we eat, where it's from, how it is made and what it contains. Which substances are we eating that we don't really know about? Many additives are chemically produced and can be modified and manipulated to produce the results that the manufacturer requires. These products can, for example, be given a longer shelf life or can be manipulated in such a way that they do not need refrigeration.

In today's world we do not prioritise planning, shopping or preparing food. Everything must be quick and time effective. Increasingly we are ordering food deliveries so that we don't even have to go to the grocery store to do the shopping ourselves and fast foods are used daily by millions of families.

Many people think that good, natural and organic foods are too expensive but looking back just a few years, we spent very little of our income on food.

Vitamins, minerals and antioxidants

Vitamins are nutrients that are necessary for our bodies to function normally. Most vitamins, minerals and antioxidants cannot be produced by our bodies and are found naturally in the foods we eat. They are a necessity. Besides providing nourishment they are necessary for the body's metabolism. Vitamin D is absorbed from the sun's rays, but all the other vitamins come from the food we eat.

The best thing is to eat a healthy combination of a variety of foods, which will provide our bodies with whatever nutrients we need. In this way you will seldom need to take extra supplements of vitamins, minerals and antioxidants.

Water-soluble vitamins

Water-soluble vitamins are vitamins that dissolve in water. Our bodies cannot store these vitamins, which means it's easier to have a deficiency, and an excess passes right through the body and is excreted when we urinate. We therefore need to eat foods that are high in water-soluble vitamins regularly.

Water-soluble vitamins are: vitamins B (1, 2, 3, 5, 6, 9, 12) and C.

Fat-soluble vitamins

Fat-soluble vitamins need fats from the foods we eat in order for our bodies to be able to absorb these vitamins. If your diet is mainly made up of carbohydrates, your body will first burn the carbs before burning fat. We need to eat fat so that our bodies can benefit from these vitamins. If your diet is low in fat, your body will not be able to absorb these vitamins and they will pass right through the bowel. Fats are a necessity.

Fat-soluble vitamins are: vitamins A, D, E and K.

Minerals

Minerals are elements and are necessary in order for our bodies to function properly. Many of the modern foods we buy have lost their natural minerals because the minerals in the soil that is used for growing have been depleted. Meat from wild animals (venison), organic and biodynamic vegetables contain more minerals than other foods.

Minerals are: iodine, iron, calcium, potassium, chromium, magnesium, manganese, sodium, selenium and zinc.

Antioxidants

Antioxidants is a collective name for substances that protect our bodies from free radicals. Free radicals can cause cholesterol to become rancid, which has a negative effect and causes heart problems.

Smoking and excess sugar in the blood increases the amount of free radicals. White sugar (sucrose) increases the speed of ageing and is closely related to the risk of cancer.

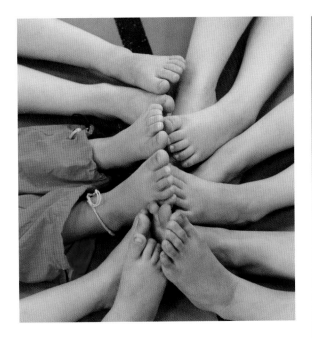

Antioxidants are found naturally in the food we eat, in particular: mushrooms, onions, berries, brightly coloured vegetables, broccoli, cabbage and cabbage-like vegetables. You will also find antioxidants in green tea, red tea (rooibos) and in dark chocolate with a high percentage of cocoa. Through eating good and natural foods we provide the body with the best way to obtain antioxidants.

Supplements

If you suspect a deficiency of any mineral, vitamin or antioxidant, then you should consider a supplement. In most cases you can read about which deficiency you may have and will recognise the symptoms that determine the deficiency. You can also do various tests by consulting your doctor.

Vitamin D

Vitamin D is necessary for the absorption of calcium and phosphorus for the growth and strength of teeth and bones. It is produced when your skin is directly exposed to the sun (UVB). In the northern hemisphere vitamin D is the most common supplement taken. In Finland, for example, children are given a vitamin D supplement until the age of 18. Adults, children and teenagers should take vitamin D supplements during winter.

Omega-3 and omega-6

Both omega-3 and omega-6 are essential, but we tend to take in too much omega-6 in comparison to omega-3. Ideally we should have a 1:1 ratio or, at most, 1:3 omega-3 and omega-6.

Oils such as corn oil, sunflower oil and margarines are usually very rich in omega-6. Too much omega-6 can cause inflammation and increase joint aches and pains.

Omega-3 plays a vital role in the development of a foetus's central nervous system and is therefore important during pregnancy. Omega-3 reduces the effects of omega-6 and protects against blood clots, eye disease and dementia. It also protects against heart disease, high blood pressure and arrhythmia, as well as stiff and painful joints. Omega-3 protects the skin against pigmentation, and improves skin conditions such as dry skin, dandruff and eczema.

Omega-3 also helps against depression and mood swings, and has an anti-inflammatory effect. In children, an omega-3 supplement has been shown to improve learning difficulties, dyslexia, concentration disability and ADHD.

We should all increase our intake of omega-3, particularly children. A good source of omega-3 is fatty fish, such as salmon, mackerel and herring. It is difficult for the body to absorb the necessary amount of omega-3 from vegetables and greens because only a small amount is converted.

If you eat fatty fish 3–5 days a week you won't need any omega-3 supplements, but if you do buy omega-3 supplements for your child, then make sure it's not with added omega-6!

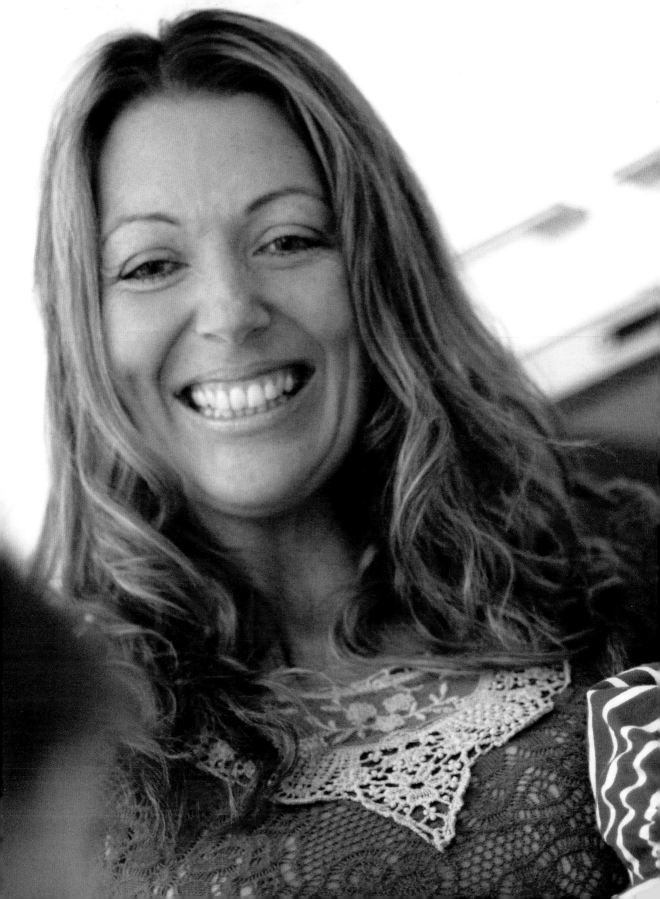

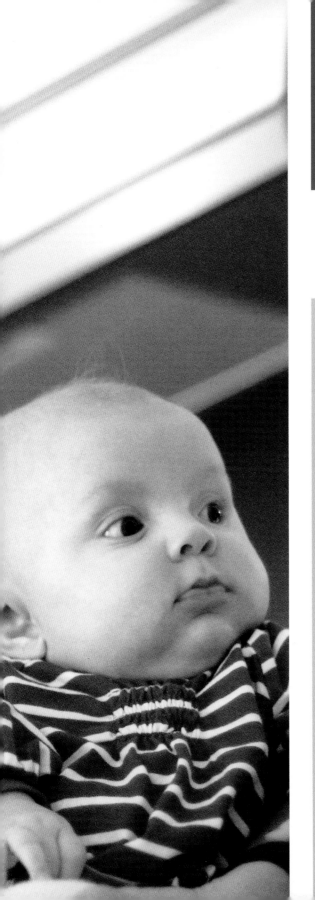

Food for babies

Breast-feeding is the natural form of feeding a baby and is also the most obvious way to nourish a newborn child. Up to the age of six months, breast milk contains all the nourishment the baby needs. From six months you can start to introduce solids, but it is advantageous to continue breast-feeding as well. Not all moms are able to breast-feed and if this is the case, the child can be given a breast milk substitute during the first six months.

As far as we can determine, during the Stone Age humans ate whatever was available, and babies and children ate more or less the same as their parents. Mothers breast-fed their children up to the age of 3 or 4 years, gradually introducing solids. Prior to the discovery of agriculture, foods such as formula, porridge, puréed fruits and sweet desserts did not exist.

Breast milk contains more than 50% energy from fat. When weaning a child off breast milk, you should gradually introduce a diet rich in fat and puréed vegetables, with lots of added fat. This is a good way to start. Avocado is a wonderful fruit that is both easy to prepare and to feed the baby. Shortly after introducing vegetables you can start to introduce foods such as liver, lamb, chicken, fish and meat, also with lots of extra fat (butter, coconut oil or ghee).

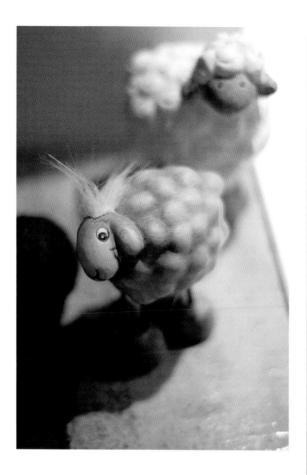

Suitable liquids

Water is the most natural source of liquid. Juice and soft drinks contain loads of sugar, which no one needs, and I do not recommend formula once the baby begins eating solids. The main ingredients in formula are flour and water or milk, and my experience shows that children who have been raised on formula after the age of 8–10 months are often very choosy or refuse to eat as they get older.

Children drink when they are thirsty, so be patient. Your child will both eat and drink when he or she needs to.

Formula substitutes

Parents often ask me what they should give their child instead of formula. I always reply: food! A child will be satisfied and fulfilled by eating natural food. If, however, a parent chooses to give their child formula, then it is important to read the label and choose the formula that is best suited to your child's needs. Many brands of formula contain maltodextrin, which is a fast-acting carbohydrate that gives a carb quick fix (turbo energy). Maltodextrin is one of the main ingredients in weight-gain solutions and in supplements that elite trainers consume after intensive training. Why is maltodextrin added to formula? Is it because it's addictive and the child will want more, and because the child experiences a 'good feeling'? Or is it for some other reason? Formula contains loads of carbohydrates and also affects the child's teeth (sugar is never good for teeth).

Food that has a higher amount of fat and less carbs will give the child energy, keep them satisfied and sustain normal weight. LCHF suits children, adults and pregnant and breast-feeding women. It is not a weight-loss programme but a lifestyle with many benefits, one of which is weight loss.

Children don't need to eat as few carbs as possible, but should eat the amount of carbs that are suited to their individual needs and tolerance. You should adjust the food and its contents to suit your children and their needs. Children that are over-active or have difficulty concentrating will benefit from eating a diet low in carbs. Remember carbs are not essential, but protein and fat are.

Many adults are already eating low carb, and there is an increasing amount of parents who choose to feed their children low-carb foods as well. These parents make conscious choices on what foods to eat and give their children, providing a healthy lifestyle. Awareness is key.

Children need nourishing foods in order to grow into healthy teenagers and adults. The right food will keep the child happy, alert and healthy. If you have a child that is overweight, low carb will also help, but consult your physician first.

Tips and foods for the first year

At around six months of age it is time to introduce a child to solids so that he or she can get used to foods that are not in liquid form. In the beginning, you can blend the food with breast milk to slowly help the child get used to new tastes and flavours.

Introduce one kind of food at a time. In this way it is easy to detect whether the child reacts to something they eat or if they have an allergy. Start off with foods that are not generally known to cause allergic reactions, for example meat, liver, chicken, butter, ghee, cold-pressed and unrefined oil, organic coconut oil, avocado and vegetables. Small tummies can be sensitive to wholewheat foods, so avoid these as your child should obtain enough fibre from vegetables. Fat is of great importance for the young child, but even for older children. There is no harm in delaying introduction of fruit purées, as these contain mostly sugars (fructose).

Introduce finger foods early so that the child will get used to new tastes and smells and also the new texture of foods. A large carrot, for instance, is great for the little one to play with and taste. At the same time the child trains hand and eye coordination and development with the muscles in the mouth.

Make sure that the finger food is large enough so that there is no risk of swallowing or choking. When children are eating they should, at all times, be supervised. Keep an eye on them once they start to get teeth to make sure they cannot bite off a piece of the food they are holding.

Always give the child dairy products high in fat instead of low- or fat-free products. You can mix heavy cream with dairy products such as yoghurt or milk.

Foods to avoid during the first year

Salt: A baby's kidneys are not developed enough to handle salt.

Fried food: Fried foods can have hard fried edges, which can be difficult to digest.

Honey: There can be traces of spores in honey that can lead to bacterial infection in the tummy.

Spinach, beetroot, and leafy celery: These contain nitrate, which can convert into nitrite in the blood. This affects oxygen uptake.

Soft cheese, such as Brie or Camembert, and liver pâté: These products contain bacteria and can cause food poisoning.

Sugar and sweeteners: All products containing sugar or sweeteners are to be avoided.

Wait until the age of 10–12 months before introducing milk, yoghurt and egg whites.

Foods that can cause allergies
Introduce these after the age of one year.

- Citrus fruit
- Shellfish
- Grains (including cereals) containing gluten, and legumes
- Strawberries

Puréed vegetables

Choose one type of vegetable at a time to see how your baby reacts:

- Turnip
- Parsnip
- Zucchini
- Carrot
- Butternut (although quite sweet)

Peel and chop the vegetable into small pieces. Place the vegetables in a saucepan and add water so that the vegetables are just covered. Cover with a lid and boil the vegetables (the nutrients and vitamins don't disappear with the steam).

Pour off the water and add some breast milk or unsalted butter (10 ml butter to 100 ml purée). Blend until smooth.

Once your little one has been eating solids for a few weeks, you can start to spice the food with fresh herbs and spices: dill, parsley, basil, thyme, coriander, ginger, tarragon, etc.

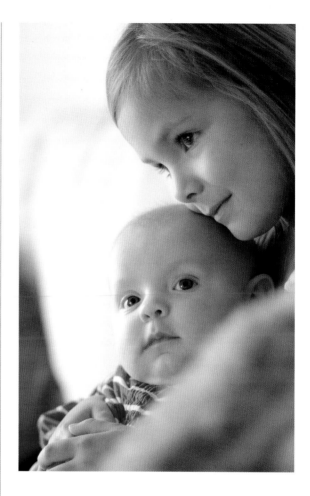

When your child has tried various vegetables, it's time to add other ingredients such as meat, chicken, potatoes, cabbage and broccoli. You can also add an egg yolk to the meal, as it is full of nutrients and filling. Only add the yolk at first, as those who are allergic to eggs are allergic to the white of the egg. Wherever possible, use organic eggs.

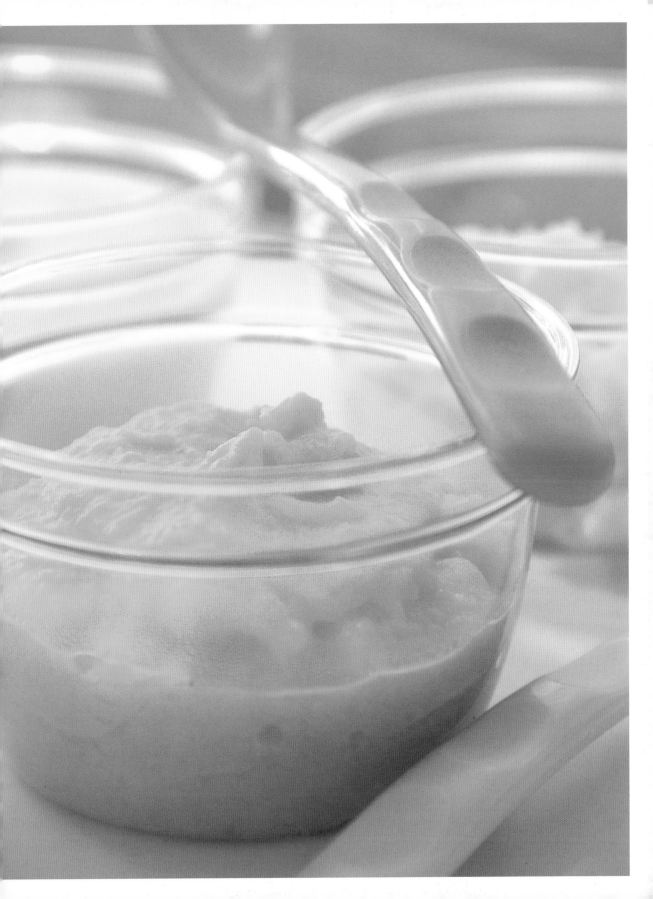

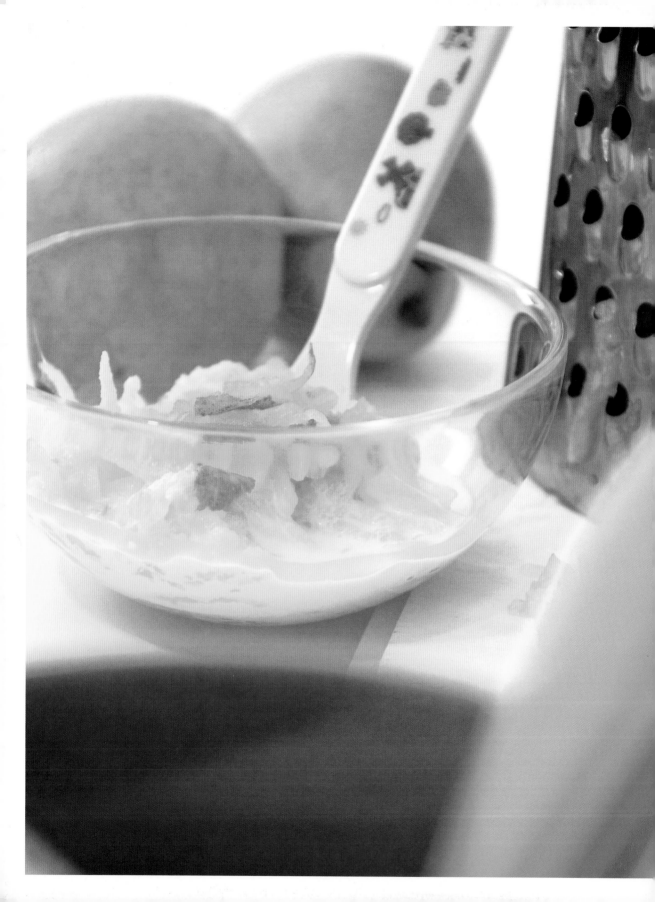

Introduce your child to drinking from a real glass at an early age. You will be surprised at how quickly they learn. Use a 'doll's size' glass for small fingers to wrap around and add only a small amount of water. At first there will be some messing but they will soon learn the technique. Provide water to drink at all times. Avoid juice and all other sweet beverages.

Foods to introduce at this age
(mash or chop the food finely)

- Fish
- Shellfish
- Unsalted nut butter (except if there are nut allergies in the family)
- Yoghurt (natural full fat)
- Cheese
- Use cream in the food
- Egg yolks

To make an egg and vegetable omelette, use vegetables that you have previously cooked and mash together with egg yolk. Fry in butter or coconut oil.

If you wish, you can add small amounts of fruit after the meal, but preferably at the same time as mealtime.

Fruit purée
Peel and chop fruit such as apple, pear or nectarine. Place the fruit in a saucepan and add a little water to cover. Cover with a lid and bring to the boil. Remove from the heat and use a hand blender or fork to mash the fruit pulp. You can even add cinnamon or cardamom while the fruit is boiling.

Fresh fruit
Peel the fruit and use a hand blender to purée the fruit in a bowl.

Pieces of fresh fruit
Peel the fruit and grate the fruit with a cheese grater. From 10–12 months you can add some heavy cream to provide extra fat and more taste.

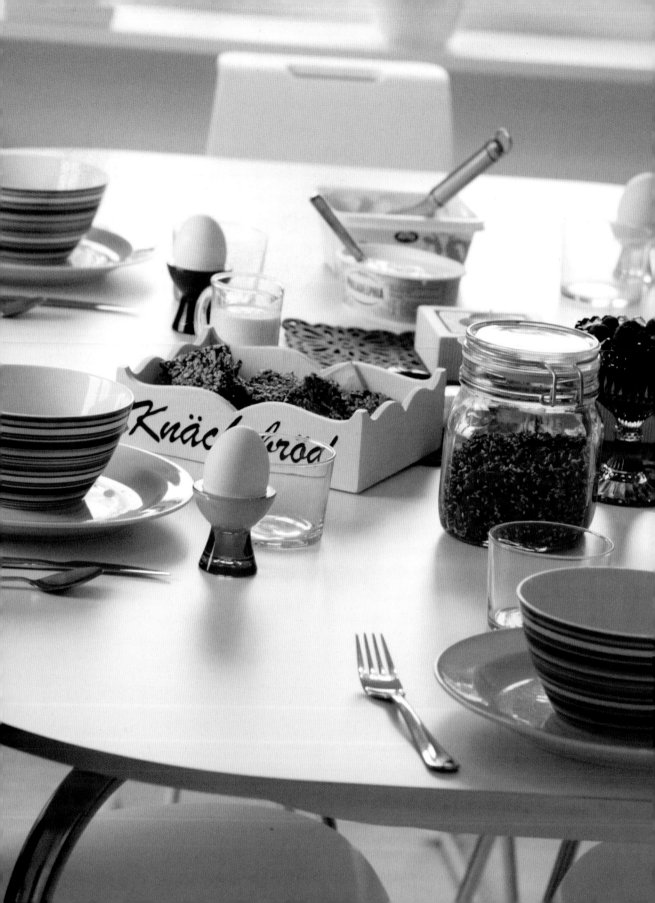

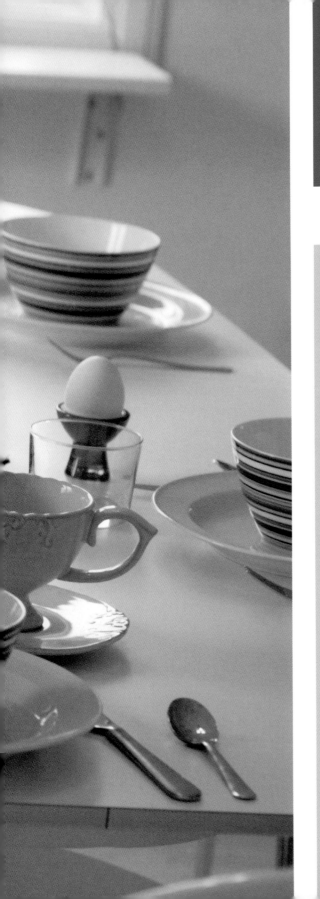

Breakfast

We have all heard that breakfast is the most important meal of the day, but what is the ideal time for breakfast? Not all people are breakfast people, and many have difficulty eating a big breakfast early in the morning. The same applies to children and teenagers.

If school mornings are not a mad rush and everyone is up and ready well before school, then there is more time to sit and enjoy the meal and everyone can eat a good and proper breakfast.

Mealtimes should be a family moment that is enjoyable. I always try to avoid nagging where food is concerned so if your children refuse breakfast, rather send them to school with something for them to eat later. Encourage your children to taste everything, but don't demand that they eat up or bribe them to finish their food. Instead, encourage your children to eat as they need nourishment and energy.

A child eats when hungry and stops eating when full. Children seldom overeat. Respect your children when they say they are full or if there is something they don't like. Are there alternatives? Ask yourself what is reasonable. You know your child best, you know what they like or don't like, and you know what they need. Make each mealtime a positive experience and remember to add variation.

Omelette
– basic recipe
1 serving

15 ml organic coconut oil or butter
2 eggs
30 ml heavy cream (whipping cream)
Salt and pepper
Extra 15 ml butter

Melt the oil or butter in a frying pan. Whisk the eggs and cream in a bowl. Add salt and pepper. Pour the mixture into the pan and fry over medium heat until the omelette has set. Turn over and fry the other side.

Serve with the extra butter on top.

Cheese omelette

Make an omelette according to the basic recipe. When one side is ready, lay 3–4 slices hard cheese (Cheddar, Gouda, etc.) or Brie cheese on half of the omelette. Fold over the other half and allow the cheese to melt over low heat.

Serve with extra butter on top.

VARIATIONS

Bacon and mushroom

Melt coconut oil or butter in a frying pan. Dice 2 rashers of bacon and slice 2 mushrooms and fry these until cooked to your liking. Mix into the basic omelette mixture and cook as described (see left).

Avocado, salami and Brie cheese

Make an omelette according to the basic recipe. When one side is ready, lay 3–4 slices salami, half a sliced avocado and some pieces of Brie cheese on half of the omelette. Fold over the other half and allow the cheese to melt over low heat.

TIPS

- Choose any of your favourite ingredients as a filling for your omelette. Fresh spinach is lovely, as is onion, Philadelphia® cream cheese or other cheese, leftover meat or sausage, pieces of cooked chicken, mayonnaise, and leeks.
- If you prefer a 'sweeter' omelette (kids usually like this), add some cinnamon to the basic mixture and serve with whipped cream and fresh berries.

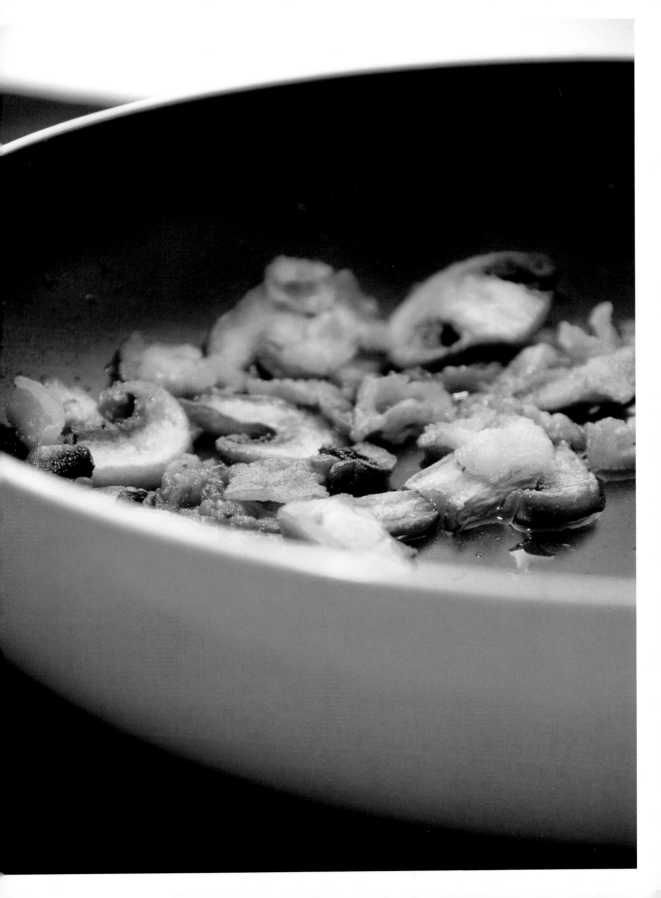

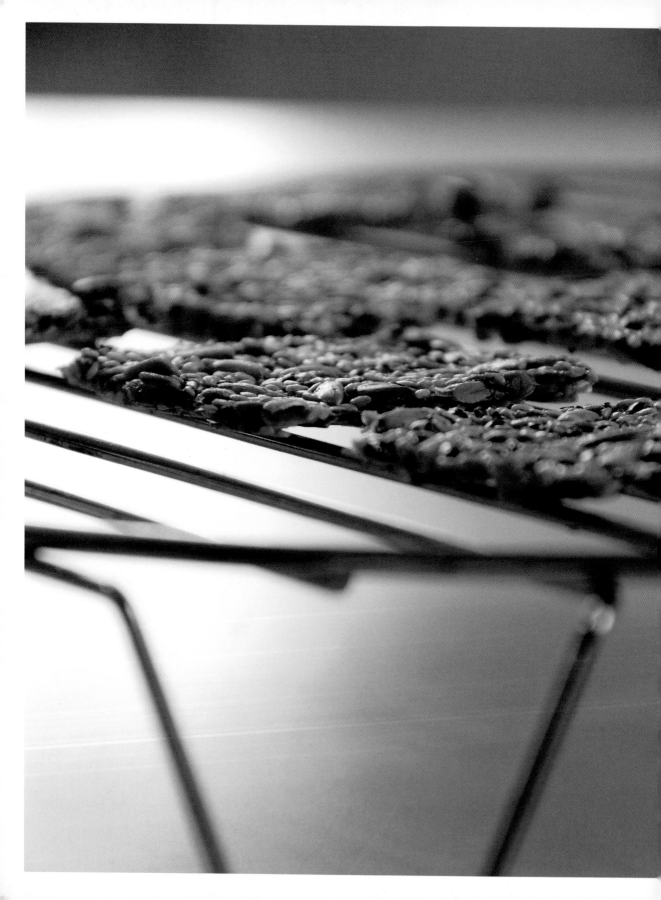

Low-carb crisp bread

Makes 16–32 pieces

200 g sunflower seeds
60 g flaxseeds
100 g sesame seeds
45 ml psyllium husk (available
  from health stores)
Pinch of salt
500 ml water

Preheat the oven to 160 °C.

Mix all the ingredients together and allow to swell for
10 minutes.

Spread the mixture on a baking sheet or 2 oven trays.
Score lines with a knife to the size you would like the
bread to be. It also makes them easier to break apart.
Bake for around 1 hour and 15 minutes.

Crisp bread breakfast

1 serving

Spread 2–3 slices low-carb crisp bread with a generous
amount of butter. Add 1–2 slices cheese of your choice
to each slice of bread. Garnish with slices of yellow
pepper, cucumber or tomato.

TIP
Remember to pre-slice the crisp
bread prior to baking it in the oven.
If you do forget, you can break it up
afterwards. It will still taste good,
but it won't have straight edges.

Low-carb muesli (cereal)

Makes 1 large batch (around 20 servings)

150 ml sesame seeds
150 ml flaxseeds
100 ml pumpkin seeds
100 ml sunflower seeds
200 ml chopped mixed nuts (unsalted)
200 ml coconut flakes (available from health stores)
10 ml ground cinnamon (optional)
Seeds from ½ vanilla pod
100 ml organic coconut oil or canola oil
100 ml water

Preheat the oven to 200 °C.

Mix all the ingredients together in a large bowl and allow to stand for 15 minutes. Spread out the muesli on a baking tray and roast for 10–20 minutes, until it turns golden in colour. Allow to cool and then store in an airtight container.

Muesli breakfast

1 serving

150 ml yoghurt (Greek, Bulgarian or plain full fat)
50 ml fresh cream
100 ml low-carb muesli
100 ml raspberries or other berries (optional)

Blend the yoghurt and cream together. Add the muesli and serve with berries on top.

For extra nourishment also eat a boiled egg with mayonnaise.

TIPS

- Feel free to add, remove or change ingredients in the muesli to suit your taste.
- Kids usually love being a part of baking muesli because there's lots of measuring, pouring and stirring.

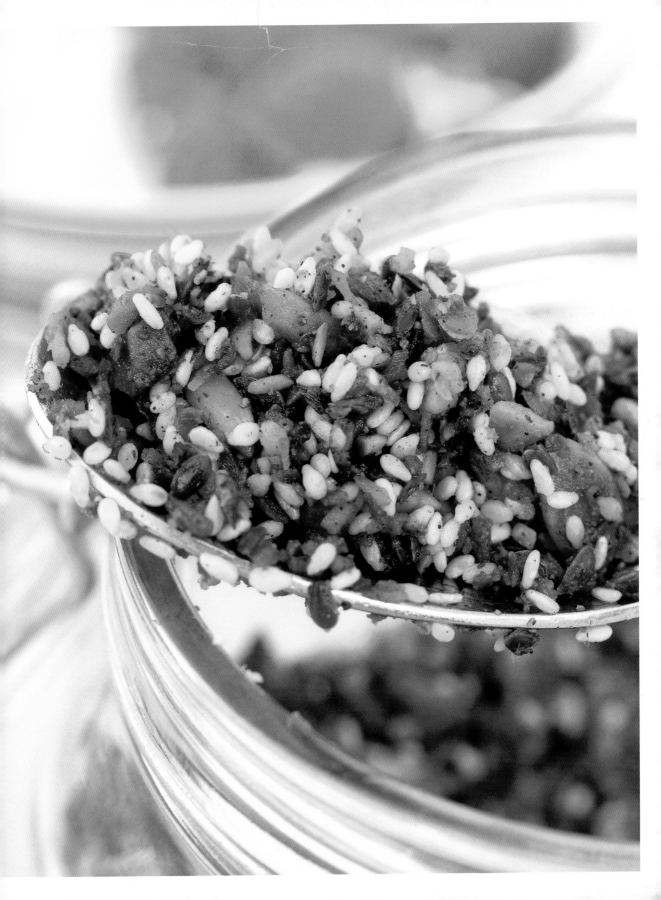

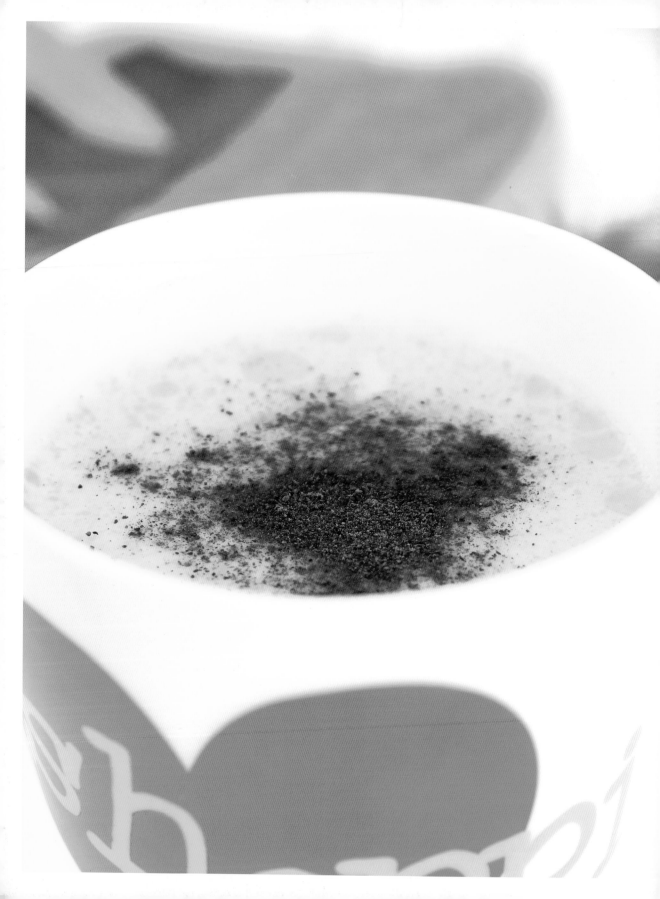

Egg milk

If you are not a breakfast person but would like something warm to drink in the morning, that also is filling, then this is a perfect beverage. It's great for children too.

1 serving

2 eggs
50 g butter or organic coconut oil
300 ml boiling water

Mix the eggs, butter or oil and water in a large mug or jug. Add a pinch of ground cinnamon or a dash of vanilla for extra flavour.

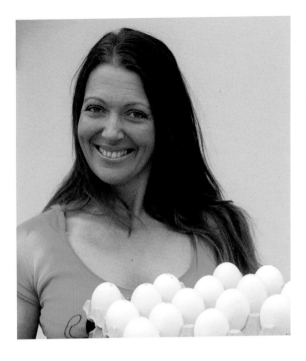

TIPS
- If you want to make hot chocolate, add 5 ml cocoa powder and seeds from ½ vanilla pod. Add 100 ml fresh cream and only 200 ml boiling water. Alternatively, melt 20 g dark chocolate and stir that into the egg milk.
- Egg milk is also a great protein drink before or after a work-out.

Creamy scrambled eggs

1 serving

15 ml organic coconut oil or butter
2 eggs
Salt and pepper
30 ml fresh cream

Melt the oil or butter in a frying pan over low heat. Mix the eggs, seasoning and cream together in a bowl. Pour the mixture into the pan. Using a spatula, scrape the eggs towards the centre of the pan. Don't overcook the eggs or they will set too firmly. Remove from the heat and serve with extra butter on top of the eggs.

TIP
For younger children (between the ages of 1 and 8 years) halve the quantities.

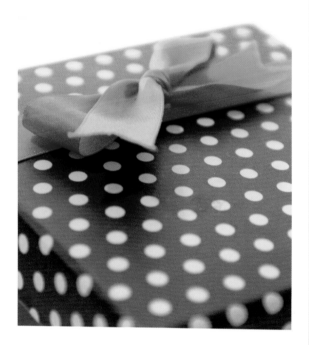

Luxury morning smoothie

1 serving

100 ml fresh cream
100 ml coconut cream (optional)
100 ml sparkling water (or natural)
100 ml yoghurt (plain)
5 ice cubes
100 ml frozen berries
4–8 almonds (optional)
Seeds from ½ vanilla pod

Mix everything together in a food processor or blender. Pour into a tall glass and enjoy.

TIP For a more filling breakfast, serve with 1 boiled egg and 15 ml mayonnaise. Smoothies also make a great snack.

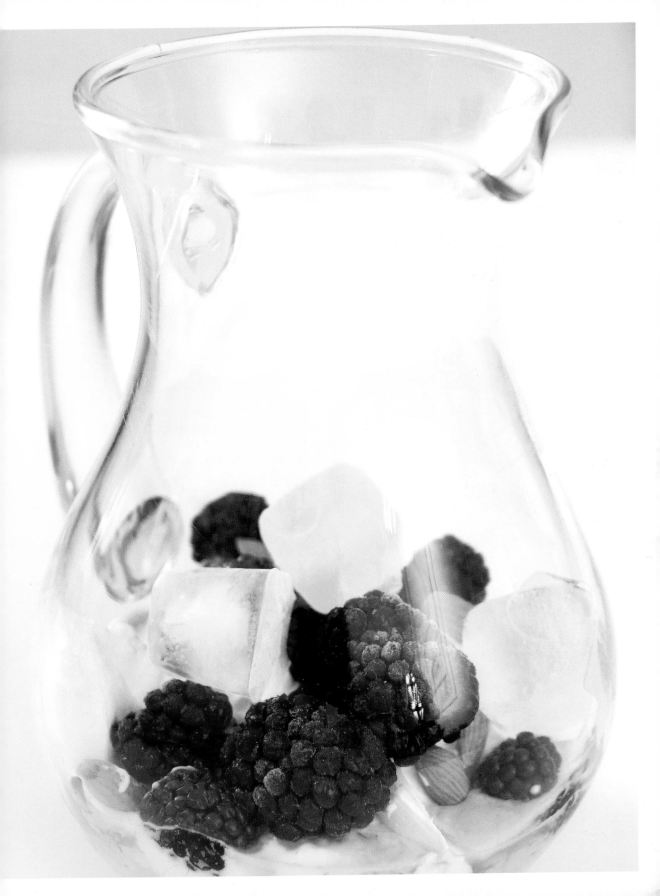

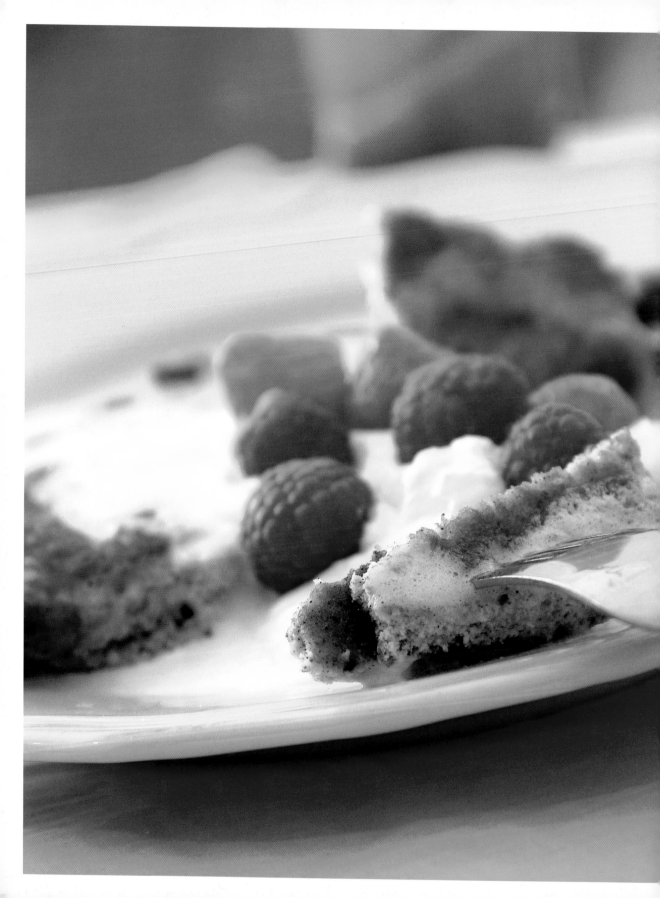

Sunday (or any day) pancake breakfast

1 serving

25 ml organic coconut oil or butter
2 eggs
100 ml fresh cream
50 ml almond flour or coconut flour (available
   from health stores)
Seeds from ½ vanilla pod
Pinch of salt
100 ml fresh cream, whipped
100 ml berries

Melt the oil or butter in a frying pan. Whisk the eggs and cream together. Add the almond or coconut flour and the vanilla and salt. Pour the mixture into the pan and fry over medium to low heat until the pancake is firm enough to turn over. Cook the other side.

Serve with whipped cream and berries.

TIP Sprinkle ground cinnamon or vanilla seeds into the whipped cream for added flavour.

Nut-free pancake

1 serving

25 ml organic coconut oil or butter
2 eggs
5 ml psyllium husk (available from health stores)
30 ml coconut flakes or coconut flour (available
   from health stores)
150 ml fresh cream
Seeds from ½ vanilla pod

Melt the oil or butter in a frying pan. Mix all the ingredients together. Pour the mixture into the pan and fry over low heat until the pancake is firm enough to turn over. Cook the other side.

Serve with whipped cream and berries, as per Sunday pancake breakfast.

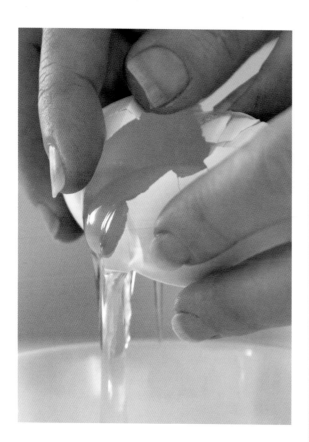

Traditional bacon and egg breakfast

1 serving

30 ml organic coconut oil or butter
3–4 rashers bacon
2 mushrooms, sliced
1 small tomato, halved (or a few cherry tomatoes)
2 eggs
30 ml mayonnaise

Melt the oil or butter in a frying pan. Fry the bacon, mushrooms and tomato until done to your liking and then remove from the frying pan. Crack the eggs and fry them in the remaining fat in the pan. Serve with mayonnaise or a knob of butter.

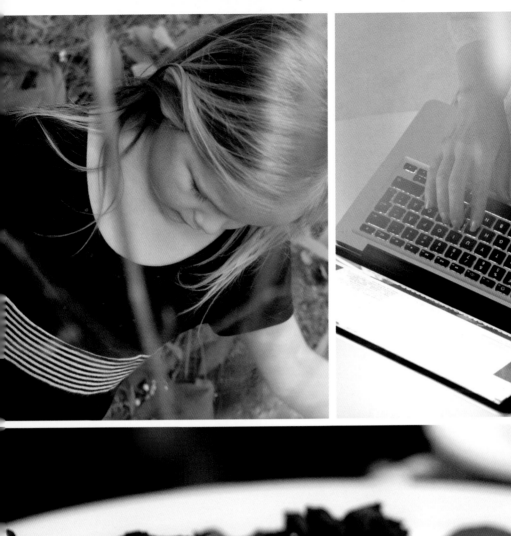

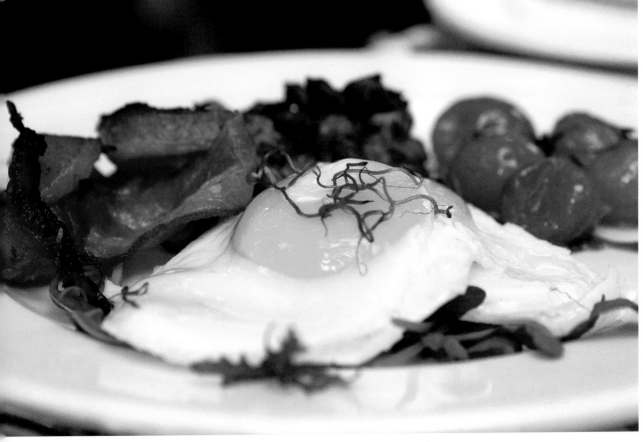

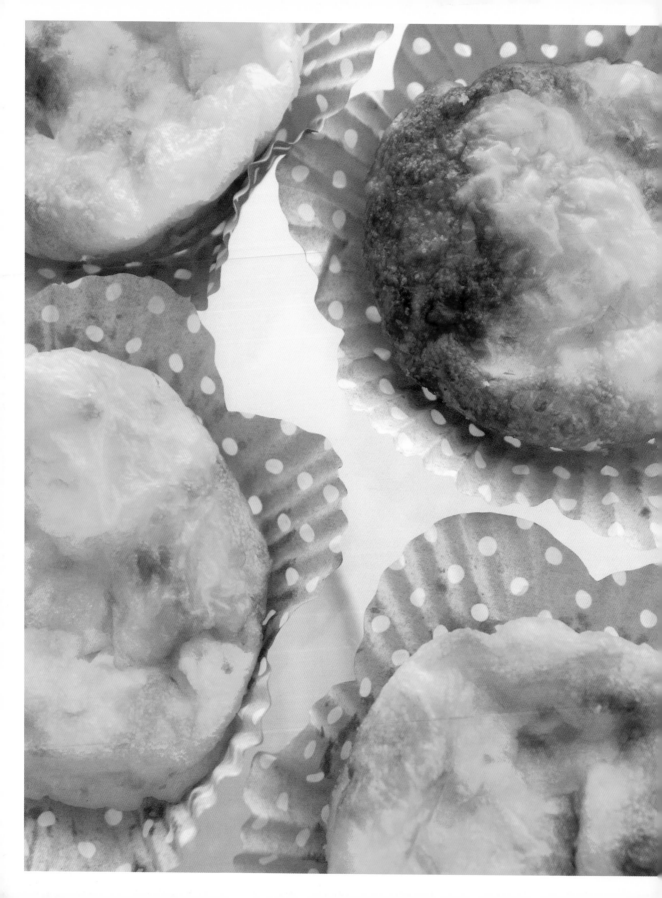

Savoury breakfast muffins

Makes 6–8 muffins

30 ml organic coconut oil or butter
4 rashers bacon, diced
½ onion, chopped
5 eggs
50 ml fresh cream
50 ml crème fraîche
Salt and pepper
Pinch of cayenne pepper
200 ml grated cheese, e.g. Cheddar

Preheat the oven to 180 °C.

Melt 15 ml of the oil or butter in a frying pan. Fry the bacon until crispy and then remove from the pan and set aside. Fry the onion until it is almost transparent.

Mix the eggs, cream, crème fraîche, seasonings and cheese together in a bowl. Stir in the bacon and onion.

Grease a muffin pan with the remaining oil or butter. Spoon the mixture into the muffin pan and bake for 20–30 minutes.

VARIATION

Reserve some of the cheese and sprinkle on top of each muffin towards the end of the baking time. This gives the muffins a lovely colour and crisp top. Keep an eye on the muffins so that the cheese does not burn.

TIPS

- These savoury muffins are great as an afternoon or late evening snack.
- You can vary the fillings with whatever ingredients you prefer, such as a small piece of Brie cheese, piquant peppers, olives, etc.

Easy 2-minute low-carb sandwich

1 serving (makes 2 breads)

1 egg
100 ml almond flour
Pinch of salt
25 ml melted butter

Beat the egg in a bowl. Add the almond flour and salt and mix together. Add the melted butter to the mixture.

Divide the mixture into two equal amounts and pour into two small bowls or dishes. Place the dishes in the microwave oven and microwave at 100% power for 2 minutes, or until you see that the bread is becoming firm and sponge-like.

Remove from the microwave and place the breads on a plate. Add lots of butter and your favourite topping: cheese and tomato, salami and Brie, ham and mustard …

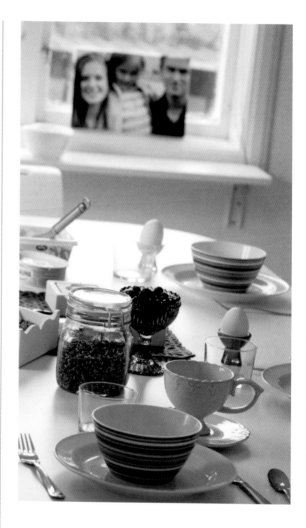

TIP The bread is quite dense and is very filling. It's also perfect to take on outings or when travelling.

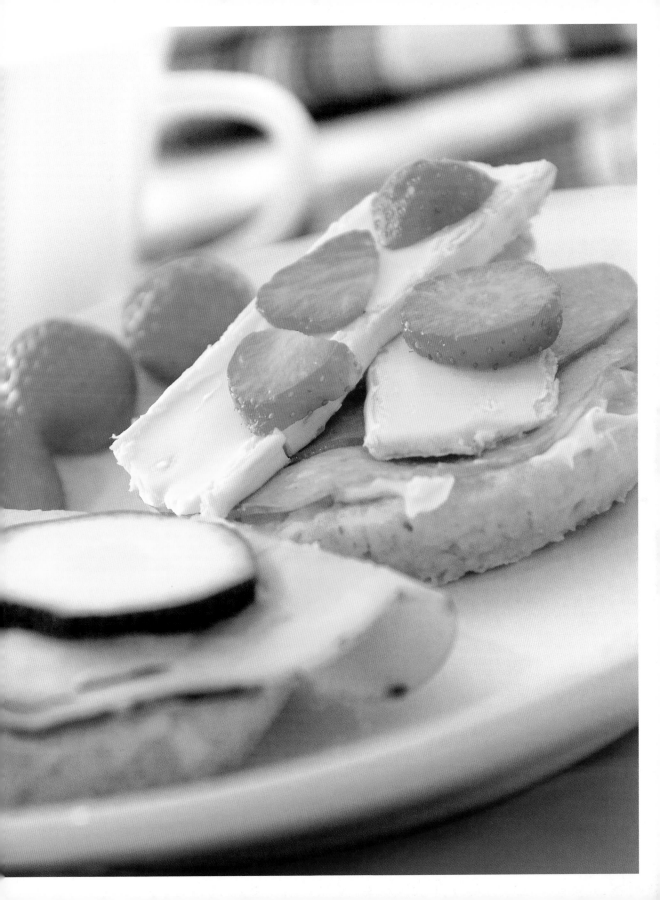

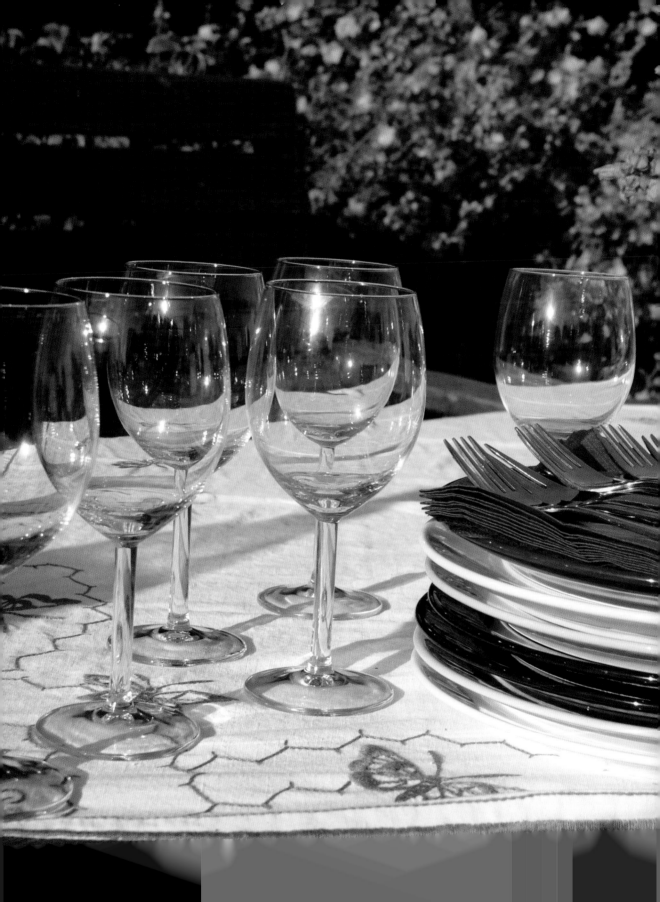

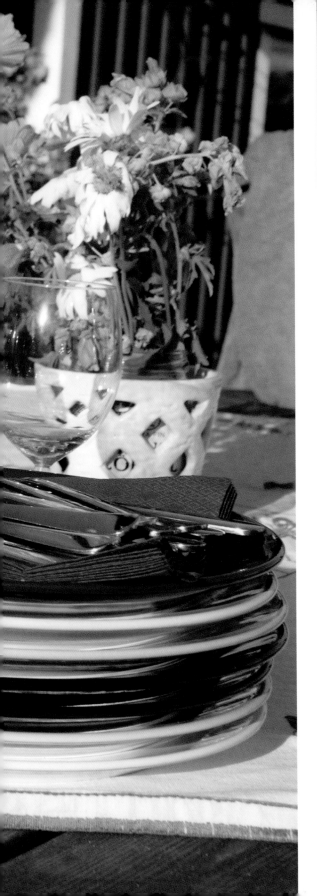

Lunch and dinner

I always put lots of effort and focus into using high-quality produce when making food. I like all the products I use to be as fresh as possible and preferably organic. When we eat produce of good quality, I believe we ingest more nourishment and less chemicals.

I emphasise the importance of avoiding processed food, and I always make meals from scratch. There are a few exceptions, such as sausage, but even then I buy only good quality with lots of meat. This also avoids the temptation of buying ready-made quick meals, which usually end up being quite expensive in the long run.

In our family we eat so that we are all full for long periods of time. This prevents cravings or the need to nibble on something constantly.

My recipes are varied so choose the ones that appeal to you and your family, for dinner or for lunch. If you make recipes in bulk you can save the leftovers for lunch the next day.

The recipes given here are easy-to-make, everyday meals and they are suitable for small children, teenagers and adults alike. All the recipes make enough for two adults and two children, unless stated otherwise.

Pork fillet with mushrooms

600 g pork fillet
Pinch of paprika
Salt and pepper
15 ml dried tarragon
5 ml ground coriander
50 g organic coconut oil or butter
4 medium mushrooms, sliced
1 onion, chopped
500 ml fresh cream
30 ml Worcestershire sauce
3 cloves garlic, crushed

Cut the fillet into 1 cm thick slices and coat with the spices (paprika, salt, pepper, tarragon, coriander). Melt half the oil or butter in a pan and fry the meat on both sides until nicely browned. Remove the meat from the pan and set aside.

Melt the rest of the oil or butter and fry the mushrooms. Add the onion and fry together with the mushrooms for around 5 minutes. Add the cream, Worcestershire sauce and garlic.

Return the meat to the pan and stir, then allow to simmer for 10 minutes.

Serve with mashed cauliflower (see page 122).

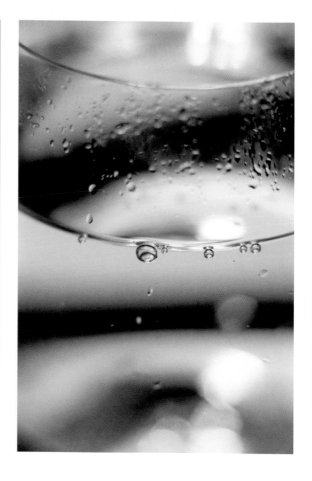

TIPS

- Coconut oil becomes liquid at 24 °C, so if the oil is in the fridge or in a cool cupboard you may need to warm it slightly in order to make it more manageable.
- Check the labels on your spice bottles to make sure they don't contain MSG. Children should not be eating anything that contains MSG!

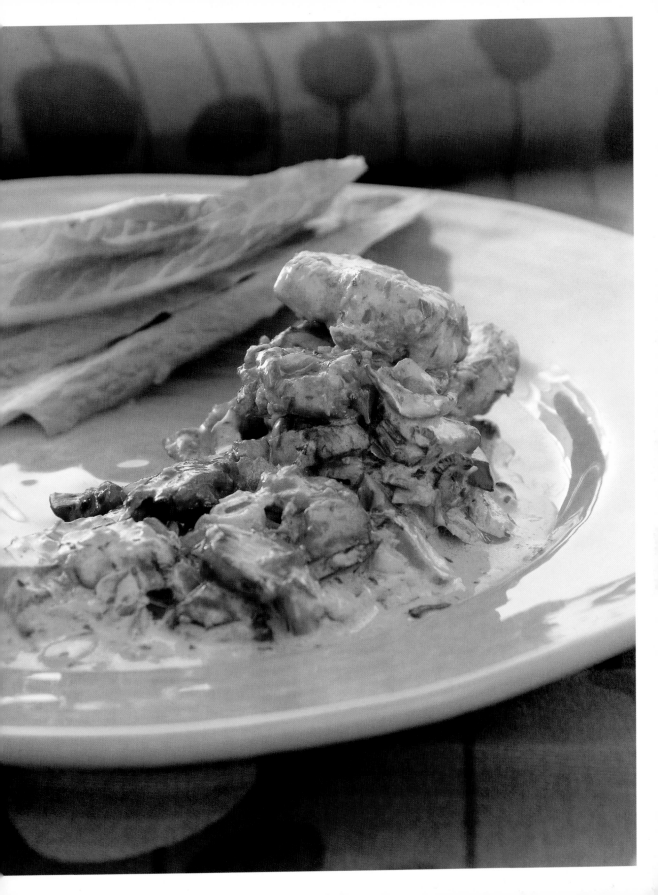

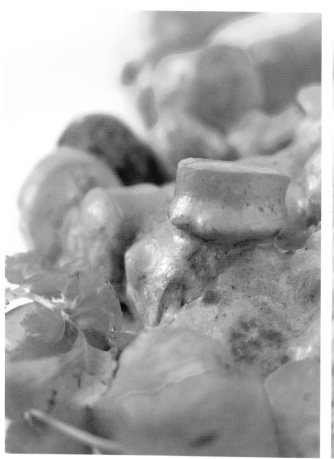
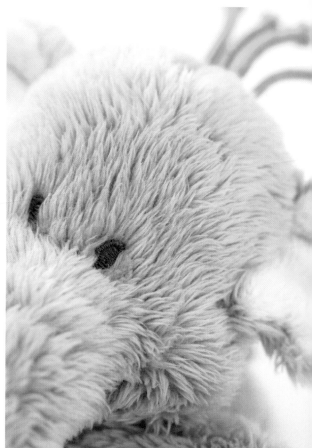
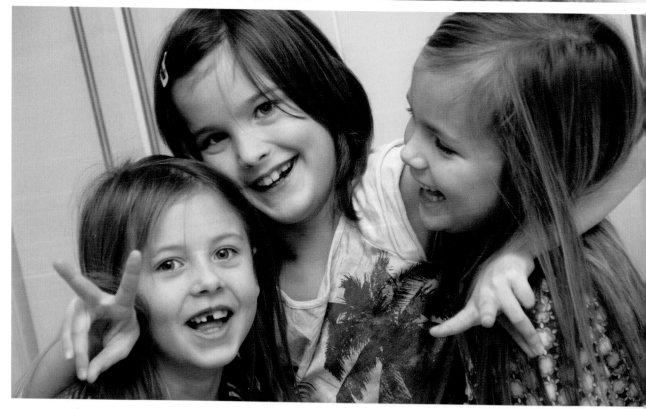

The kids' favourite stroganoff

25 ml organic coconut oil or butter
400 g sausage (at least 80% meat), diced
5 ml sea salt
10 ml paprika
Pinch of cayenne pepper
15 ml dried tarragon
2.5 ml nutmeg
500 ml fresh cream
1–2 onions, chopped
3 cloves garlic, crushed
15 ml tomato purée
30 ml Dijon mustard

Melt the oil or butter in a saucepan. Fry the sausage for a few minutes and then add the salt, spices and cream. Add the onions, garlic, tomato purée and mustard and simmer for 5–10 minutes.

Serve with boiled broccoli and salad.

TIP Dijon mustard is low in carbs and is a good alternative when adding flavour to food.

Meatballs with gravy

500 g minced meat
2 organic eggs
100 ml fresh cream
80 g chopped walnuts (optional)
30 ml chopped fresh parsley
1 onion, chopped
2 cloves garlic, crushed
10 ml ground coriander
5 ml grated nutmeg
5 ml ground ginger
10 ml sea salt
2.5 ml white pepper
2.5 ml cayenne pepper
150 g organic coconut oil or butter

Mix all the ingredients together in a large bowl, including 50 g of the coconut oil or butter.

Using around a tablespoonful of meat mixture at a time, roll the mince into balls. Melt the rest of the oil or butter in a pan and fry the meatballs, turning often, until browned all over. Alternatively, you can arrange the meatballs on a baking tray lined with greaseproof paper and then grill the meatballs in the centre of the oven for around 15 minutes, or until they start to get colour.

Gravy

300 ml fresh cream
15 ml Worcestershire sauce

Use the drippings from the frying pan when making the gravy. Strain the oil and pour into a saucepan. Add the cream and Worcestershire sauce and simmer until the gravy starts to thicken.

Serve the meatballs with mashed cauliflower (see page 122) and the gravy.

TIPS

- You can use a spoon and a cup of hot water when you roll the meatballs. Place the meat in your hand and form a ball using the spoon. Dip the spoon into the water every time so that the meat does not stick to it.
- If you want thicker gravy, remove it from the heat and add an egg yolk, stirring continuously until thickened.

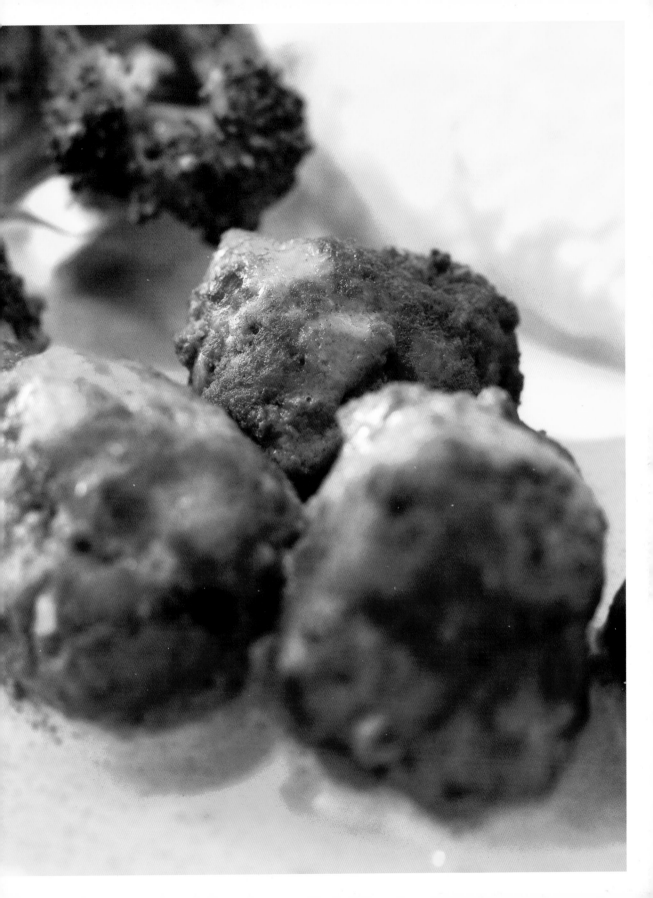

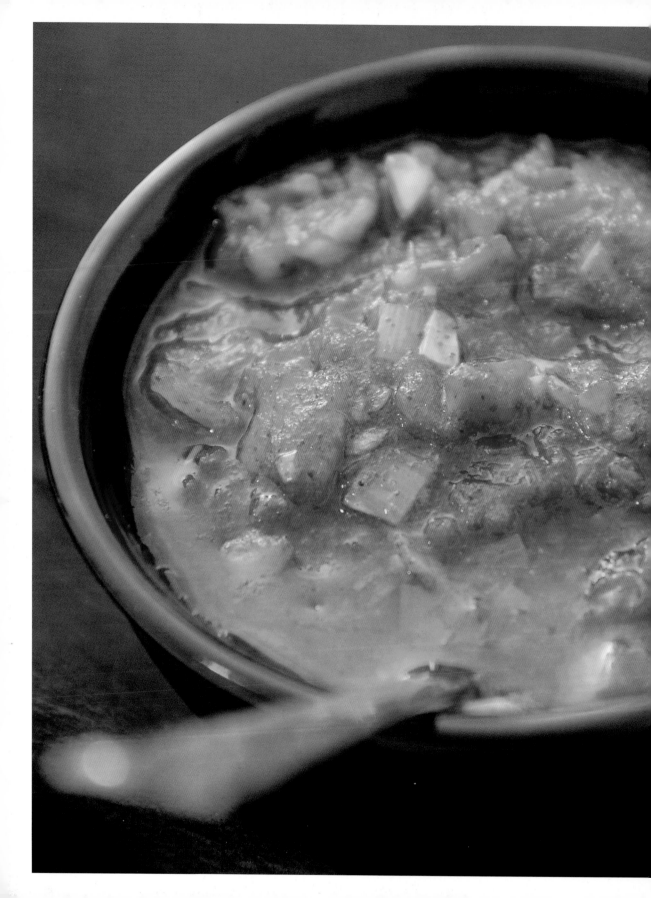

Mexican mince with taco sauce

50 g organic coconut oil or butter
500 g minced meat
3 cloves garlic, crushed
7.5 ml chilli powder or dried chilli
30 ml ground cumin
5 ml paprika
5 ml cayenne pepper
5 ml black pepper
5 ml ground cinnamon
1 yellow pepper, chopped
200 g Philadelphia® cream cheese
300 ml crème fraîche
1 onion, sliced into rings
1 tomato, thinly sliced
400 ml grated cheese

Preheat the oven to 200 °C.

Melt the oil or butter in a frying pan and fry the minced meat until browned. Add the garlic and all the spices and stir thoroughly. Add the yellow pepper and stir it into the meat.

Mix the cream cheese and crème fraîche together in a bowl. Spread this out evenly on the bottom of an ovenproof dish. Spoon the minced meat carefully over the cheese mixture and layer the onion rings and slices of tomato on top. Sprinkle with the grated cheese and bake for 20 minutes.

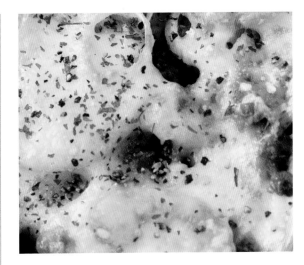

Taco sauce

3 large tomatoes
50 g butter
1 onion, chopped
5 cm-piece leek, chopped
1 red pepper, chopped
2 cloves garlic, chopped
2 jalapeño chillies, chopped
100 ml water
Salt and pepper
5 ml paprika
15 ml tomato purée
45 ml vinegar

Place the tomatoes in a saucepan and add water to cover. Boil for a few minutes, then remove the tomatoes and peel them.

Melt the butter in a saucepan. Add the tomatoes, onion, leek, red pepper, garlic and chillies and fry for a few minutes while stirring. Add the water, seasoning, paprika, tomato purée and vinegar. Simmer for 15 minutes. Remove from the heat and allow to cool.

The sauce can be made in advance and stored in the fridge for a few days.

Serve with cheese chips (see page 182) and the sauce on the side.

TIPS

- In my experience, children don't really like warm slices of tomato, so cover only half of the dish with tomatoes if you have family members that don't enjoy baked tomatoes.
- The sauce is a bit too spicy for little ones, but adults usually love it. Serve the sauce separately.

Low-carb soup

50 g organic coconut oil or butter
10 mushrooms, sliced
600 g minced meat
800 ml fresh cream
250 ml water (you can add more if the soup is
   too thick)
30 ml dried tarragon
15 ml paprika
30 ml tomato purée
Salt and pepper
2 onions, roughly chopped
50 ml chopped fresh parsley
3 cloves garlic, chopped
1 yellow pepper, chopped
100 g butter
Crème fraîche for serving

Melt the 50 g oil or butter in a pan. Fry the mushrooms
until crisp and then remove from the pan and transfer
to a separate saucepan. Fry the mince in batches, and
then add to the mushrooms. Add the cream, water,
tarragon, paprika, tomato purée and seasoning. Add
the onions and bring to the boil. Reduce the heat and
simmer for 10–15 minutes.

Add the parsley and garlic, and then add the yellow
pepper. Stir in the 100 g butter.

Serve the crème fraîche separately so everyone can
add their own.

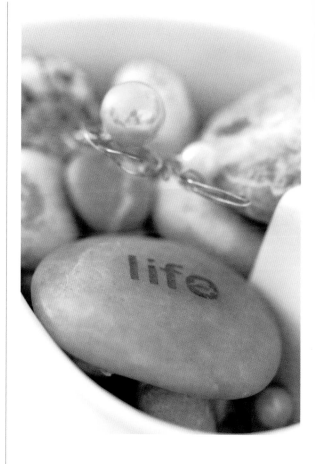

TIP
The extra butter helps enhance the
flavour of the soup and makes you
feel full.

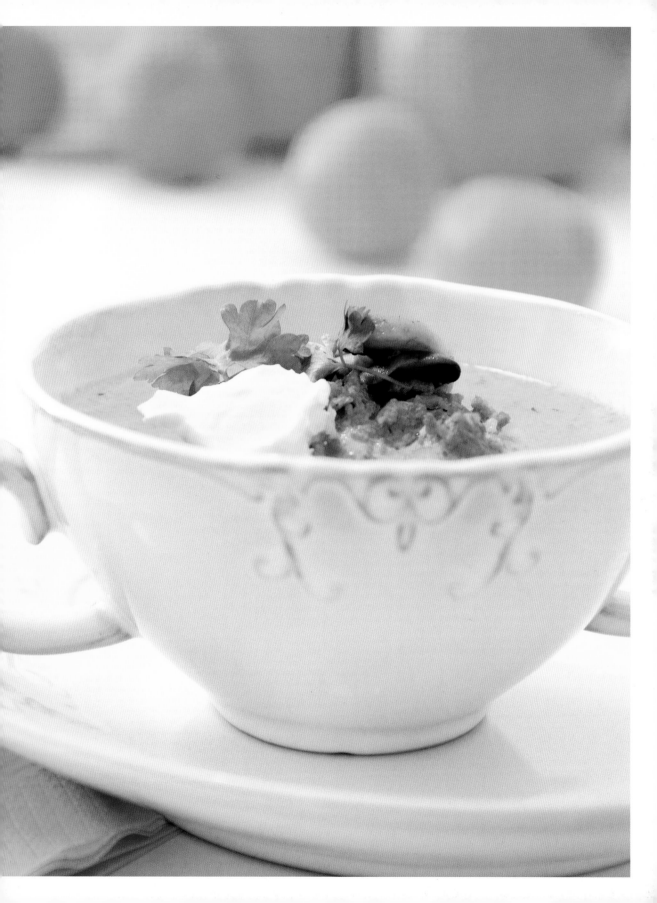

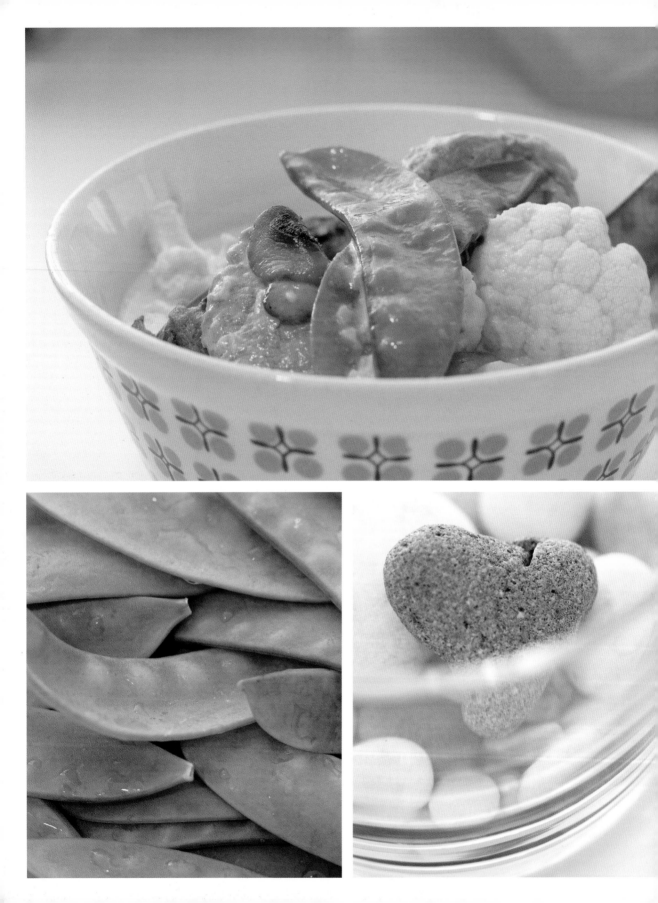

Pork fillet stew with mange tout and parsley

50 g organic coconut oil or butter
4 large mushrooms, sliced
600 g pork fillet, cut into 1 cm slices
1 red onion, chopped
⅓ head cauliflower, broken into florets
3–4 cloves garlic, crushed
200 ml fresh cream
200 ml crème fraîche
Pinch of nutmeg
Salt and pepper
Pinch of cayenne pepper
180 ml chopped fresh parsley
15 mange tout
10–15 olives

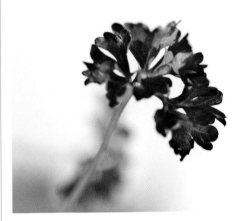

Melt the oil or butter in a pan and fry the mushrooms until crisp. Transfer the mushrooms to a separate saucepan. Brown the pork fillet in the frying pan (you may need to use more oil or butter). Add the meat to the mushrooms.

Add the onion, cauliflower and garlic and pour in the cream. Add the crème fraîche to the stew. Bring to the boil and add the spices, parsley, mange tout and olives. Simmer for 5–10 minutes.

Serve with a salad.

TIP Choose nourishing leaves for your salad, such as rocket, romaine or cos lettuce, or fresh spinach.

Thai stir-fry with ginger and coconut

50 g organic coconut oil or butter
5 mushrooms, chopped
⅓ head cauliflower, broken into florets
½ head broccoli, broken into florets
1 onion, sliced
1 leek, sliced
15 ml green curry paste
400 g chicken fillets (or minced meat)
400 ml coconut cream
200 ml fresh cream
Salt and pepper
4 cloves garlic
45 ml grated fresh ginger
Grated zest and juice of 1 lime
45 ml Philadelphia® cream cheese
1 red pepper, sliced into rings
15 ml chopped fresh coriander

 TIP Coconut cream contains more fat and less carbs than coconut milk.

Melt the coconut oil or butter in a wok and stir-fry the mushrooms, cauliflower and broccoli until cooked but still crisp. Remove the vegetables from the pan and set aside.

Add the onion, leek and curry paste to the wok and stir-fry for a couple of minutes. Cut up the chicken and add to the onion and curry paste. Add the coconut cream, fresh cream, seasoning, garlic, ginger and lime. Stir-fry for a couple of minutes until the chicken is cooked.

Add the cream cheese and stir well. Add the fried vegetables and top with red pepper rings. Serve garnished with fresh coriander.

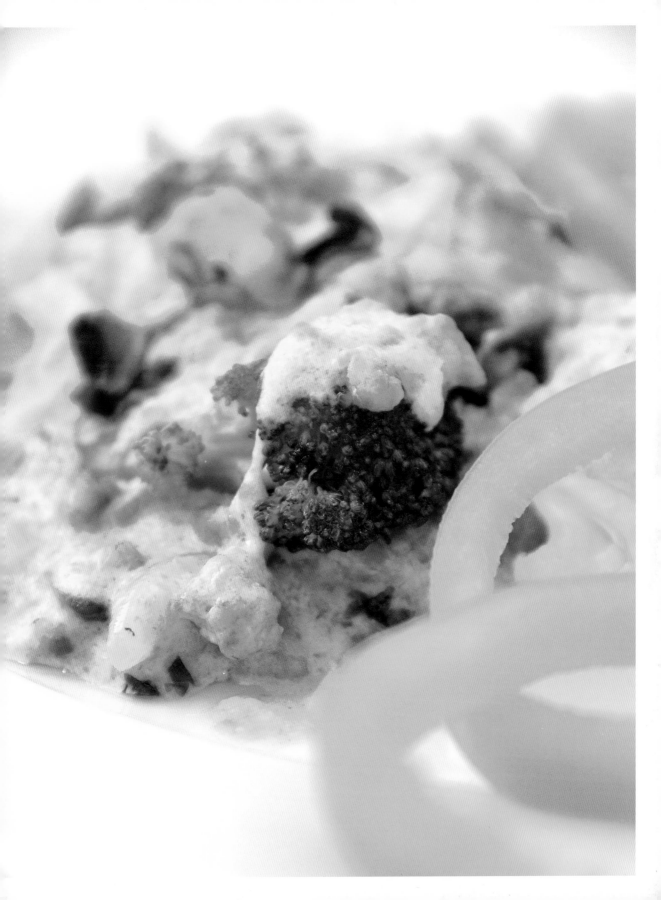

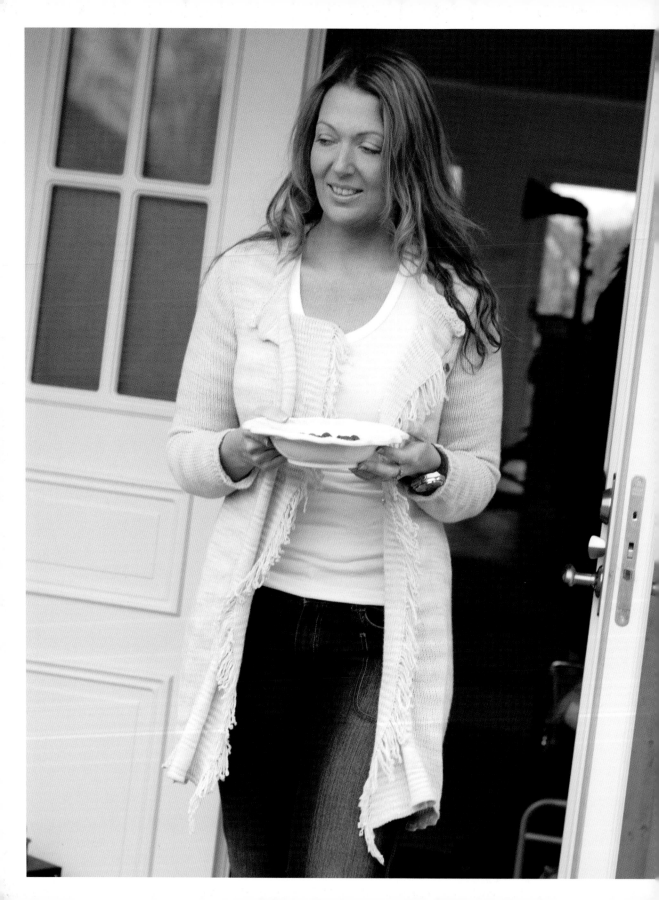

Bacon and sausage bake

250 g cauliflower, broken into florets
300 ml fresh cream
30 ml organic coconut oil or butter
250 g bacon, diced
300 g sausage (at least 80% meat), diced
1 onion, chopped
3 cloves garlic, crushed
200 ml grated Parmesan cheese

Preheat the oven to 180 °C.

Place the cauliflower and cream in a saucepan. Bring to the boil and simmer for 10 minutes.

Heat 15 ml of the oil or butter in a frying pan and fry the bacon until crisp. Remove and set aside.

Add the rest of the oil or butter to the pan and fry the sausage and the onion.

Blend the cauliflower with a hand blender until smooth. Add the bacon, sausage and onion to the cauliflower. Add the garlic and mix together.

Place the cauliflower mixture in an ovenproof dish and bake for 10–15 minutes, or until golden. Remove from the oven and sprinkle the grated Parmesan cheese on top. Set the oven on grill function and grill the dish for a few minutes until the cheese is crisp and golden.

Serve with a salad.

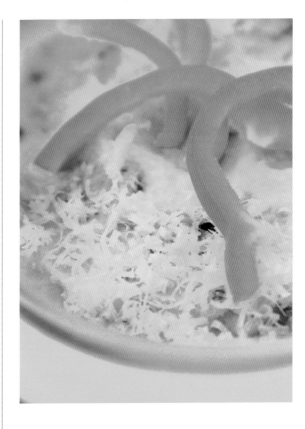

TIP

Always read the list of ingredients when buying sausage and make sure you choose one with high meat content. Aim for a meat content as close to 100% as possible.

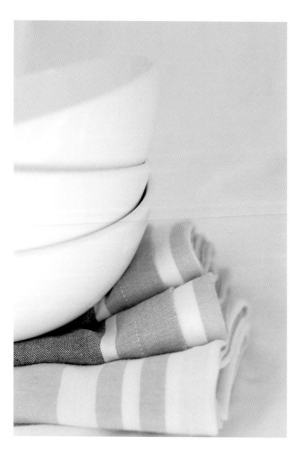

Goulash soup

30 ml organic coconut oil or butter
300 g sirloin or other cut of beef, cut into cubes
or strips
1 fennel bulb, chopped
1 onion, chopped
10 cm-piece leek, sliced
1 yellow, red or green pepper, chopped
3 cloves garlic
2.5 ml ground cumin
25 ml tomato purée
1 chilli, chopped
2.5 ml paprika
Pinch of cayenne pepper
5 medium mushrooms, sliced
700 ml water
Salt and pepper
Crème fraîche for serving

Melt half the oil or butter in a saucepan and fry the meat until it has a nice colour. Add the fennel, onion, leek and yellow pepper and fry for a couple of minutes.

Grind the garlic and cumin together using a mortar and pestle and stir in the tomato purée, chilli, paprika and cayenne pepper to form a paste. Add the paste to the meat and vegetable mixture and set aside.

Melt the rest of the oil or butter in a frying pan and fry the mushrooms until browned and crisp. Add to the meat and vegetable mixture along with the water, salt and pepper and allow to simmer for 20 minutes over moderate heat.

Serve with a heaped spoon of crème fraîche in each soup bowl.

TIP

Depending on how sensitive you are to root vegetables, you may want to add 1-2 carrots. Parboil for 5 minutes and then add them when you add the meat.

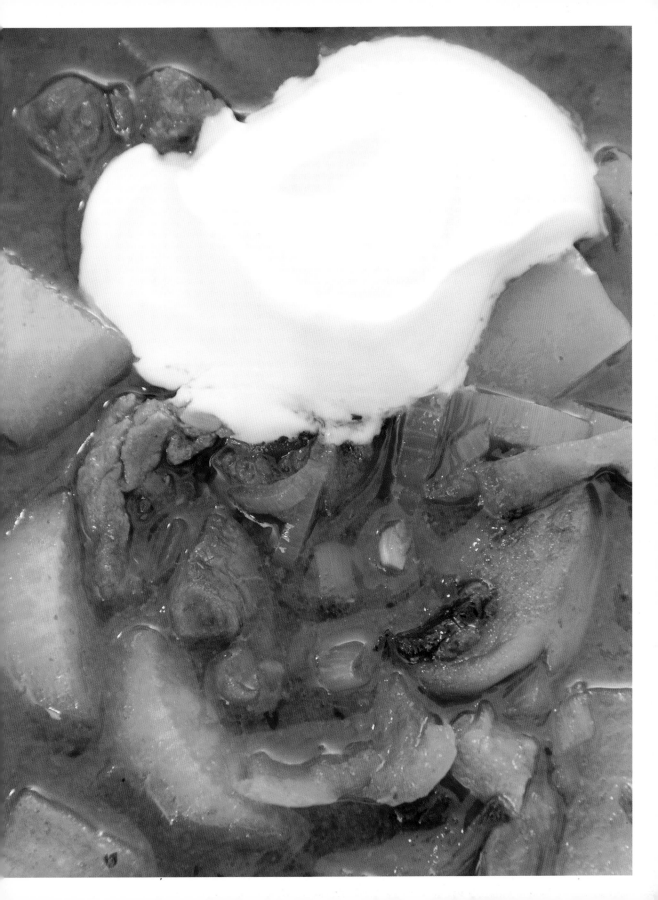

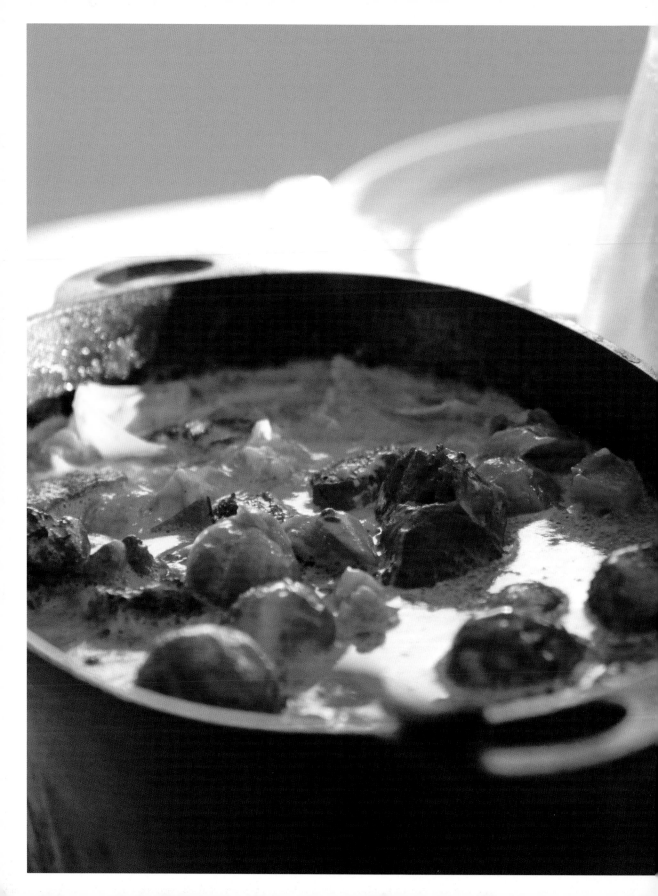

Lamb stew

100 g organic coconut oil or butter
1 kg shoulder of lamb, cut into cubes
2 litres water
Salt and white pepper
6 sun-dried tomatoes
8–10 medium mushrooms, cut into chunks
1 onion, chopped
½ leek, sliced
60–75 ml grated fresh horseradish
30 ml chopped fresh coriander
15 ml paprika
500 ml fresh cream
30 ml Dijon mustard
8–10 Brussels sprouts

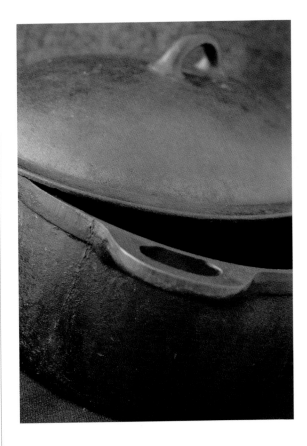

Heat half the oil or butter in a pan and brown the meat in batches. Place the fried meat in a casserole pot and add just enough of the water to cover the meat. Bring to the boil and then reduce the heat.

Add the seasoning and the sun-dried tomatoes and simmer over low heat for 3 hours. Switch off the heat and allow the meat to stand in the pot, covered, for another 2 hours.

Heat the remaining oil or butter in a pan and fry the mushrooms, onion and leek. Add them to the stew. Stir in the horseradish, coriander, paprika, cream and mustard. Add more salt and pepper if needed. Bring the stew to a simmer and add the Brussels sprouts 5 minutes before serving.

Serve with fresh tomatoes and cauliflower rice (see page 129).

TIP When you buy sun-dried tomatoes, make sure they are not in sunflower oil. If so, rather buy dried tomatoes in a bag and put them in a jar with your own choice of good oil, such as olive oil or avocado oil.

Low-carb bobotie

50 g organic coconut oil or butter
1 onion, chopped
Salt and pepper
Pinch of cayenne pepper
10 ml curry powder
2.5 ml ground cinnamon
500 g minced beef or lamb
½ apple, finely chopped
2 dried apricots, finely chopped
1 tomato, peeled and diced
75 ml flaked almonds
60 ml desiccated coconut
150 ml fresh cream
45 ml balsamic vinegar

Topping
4 eggs
200 ml fresh cream

Preheat the oven to 180 °C.

Heat the oil or butter in a large frying pan and fry the onion with all the spices. Add the meat and fry until browned. Add the rest of the ingredients and fry for a few minutes.

Spoon the meat mixture into an ovenproof dish. Beat the eggs and cream together for the topping and pour over the meat. Bake for 20–30 minutes until the egg mixture has set and the bobotie has a golden colour.

Serve the bobotie as is or with a salad.

TIP

Feel free to exclude the apricots or to add a bit more, depending on how strict you are with your eating plan. Bobotie is known to be slightly sweet and usually contains jam or raisins. In this recipe the coconut and apple add the sweetness.

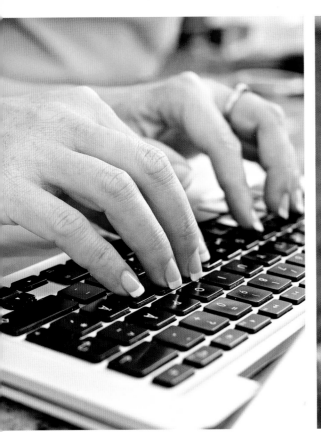
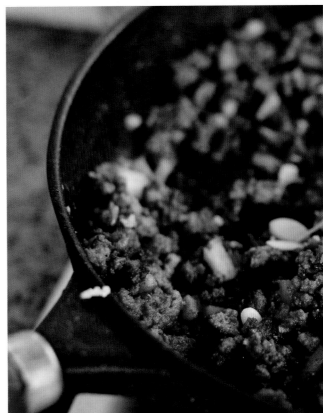
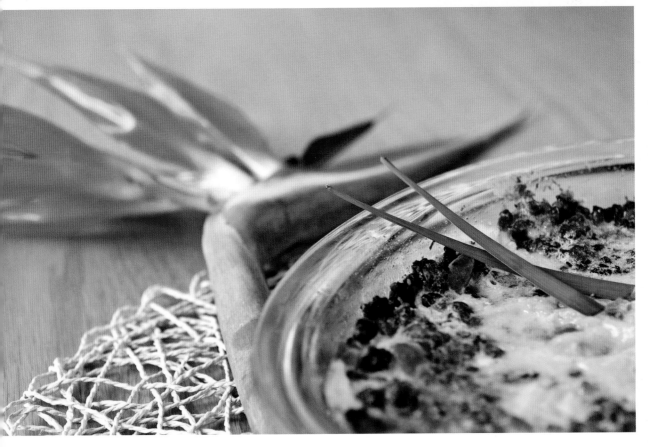

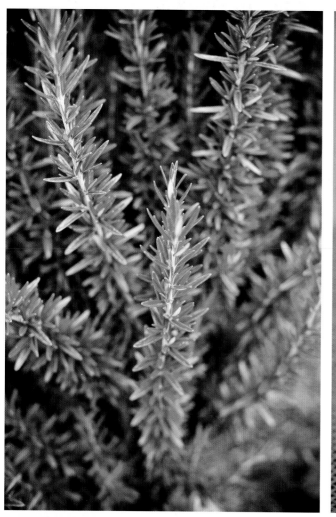
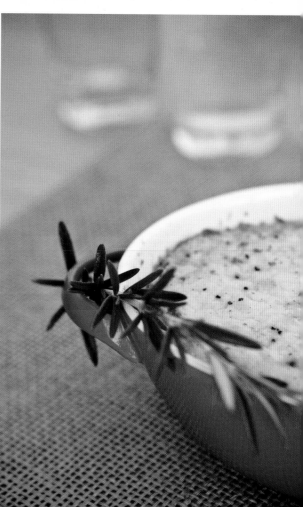
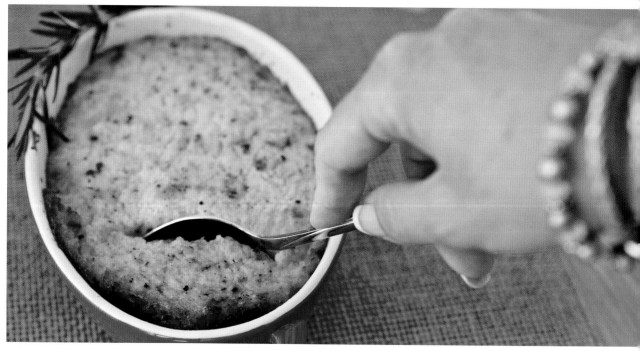

Shepherd's pie

50 g organic coconut oil or butter
2 onions, chopped
500 g minced lamb or beef
1 carrot, finely chopped
3 cloves garlic, crushed
50 g organic coconut oil or butter
1 tomato, peeled and chopped
5 ml tomato paste
45 ml Worcestershire sauce
Salt and pepper
200 ml fresh cream

Topping

1 head cauliflower
2 cloves garlic, crushed
15 ml chopped fresh parsley
Salt and pepper
100 g butter
200 ml grated Cheddar cheese
15 ml butter

Preheat the oven to 180 °C.

Heat the oil or butter in a frying pan and fry the onions. Add the mince and sauté until browned. Add the remaining ingredients and simmer for 10 minutes, stirring regularly.

Topping

Chop up the cauliflower and boil in water until soft. Drain the cauliflower and add the garlic, parsley, salt and pepper and butter. Using a hand blender, mash the cauliflower until smooth. Add the grated cheese and mix well.

Spoon the meat mixture into an ovenproof dish. Spread the cauliflower mash over the top, covering the entire dish so that it creates a seal to prevent the mixture from bubbling over when in the oven. Add the 15 ml butter to the top and then bake for 20–25 minutes, or until the cauliflower mash begin to brown.

Serve with salad.

 TIP This dish can be prepared ahead of time and baked just before serving.

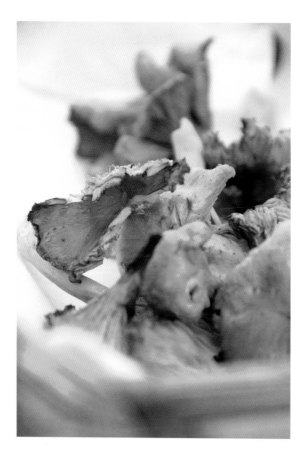

Chicken casserole with mushrooms

50 g organic coconut oil or butter
100 g dried or fresh chanterelles (or other
 mushrooms)
3–4 chicken fillets, diced
400 ml fresh cream
15 cm-piece leek, chopped
3 cloves garlic, crushed
1 onion, chopped
200 g cauliflower, broken into florets
45 ml good-quality vinegar
15 ml Dijon mustard
2 egg yolks

Melt the oil or butter in a saucepan. Add the
chanterelles or other mushrooms and fry for a few
minutes. Add the chicken and pour in the cream.

Add the leek, garlic, onion, cauliflower, vinegar
and mustard and simmer for 15 minutes, stirring
occasionally.

Add the egg yolks, one at a time, stirring continuously
until creamy and thick.

Eat as is or serve with mashed broccoli (see page 122).

Eat as is or serve with mashed broccoli (see page 122).

TIPS

- This casserole tastes great, even without the mushrooms.
- Garlic contains 31 g carbohydrates per 100 g.

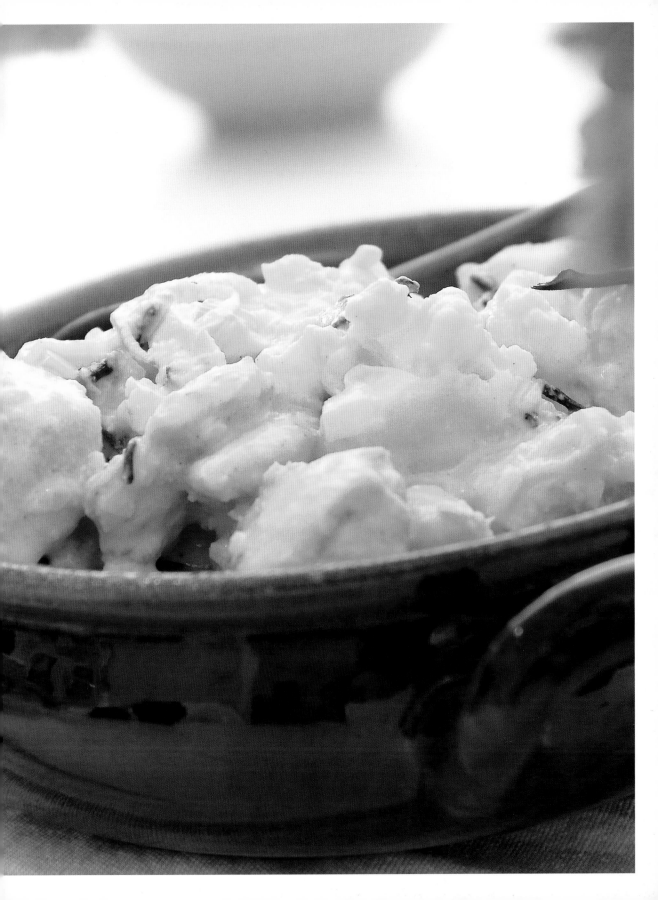

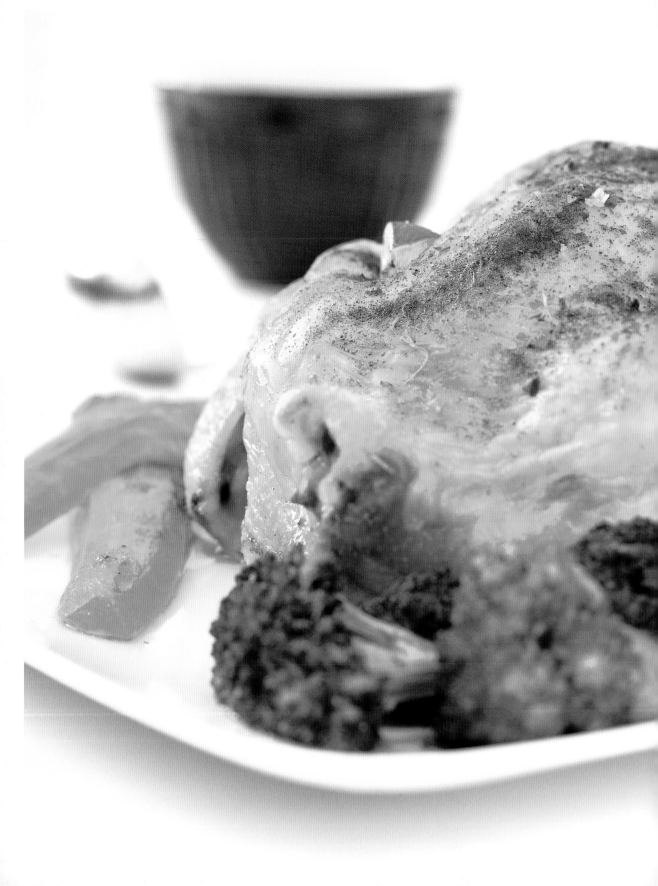

Roast chicken with lime and garlic and roasted veg

100 g organic coconut oil or butter
1 whole chicken
2 limes
30 ml dried tarragon
6 cloves garlic, peeled
5 ml cayenne pepper
5 ml paprika
5 ml ground sea salt

Vegetables

4–6 broccoli florets
1 carrot
1 baby marrow (courgette, zucchini)
1 onion
100 ml organic coconut oil (heat slightly if
    necessary to liquefy)
1 clove garlic, crushed
Salt and pepper

Preheat the oven to 180 °C. Grease an ovenproof dish or baking tray with half the oil or butter.

Rinse and dry the chicken. Cut the limes into wedges and squeeze the juice into a glass. Place the tarragon, garlic and lime wedges inside the chicken cavity. Rub the chicken with the remaining oil or butter and sprinkle with the cayenne pepper, paprika, salt and the lime juice. Place the chicken in the prepared dish.

Cut up the vegetables and place them in a small freezer bag. Add the oil, garlic and seasoning. Close the bag and shake the vegetables until they are coated with oil. Remove the vegetables from the bag and place them all around the chicken.

Roast for 45–70 minutes, depending on your oven and the size of the chicken. Near the end of the cooking time, set the oven on grill function and grill the chicken until golden and crisp.

Serve with cauliflower rice (see page 129).

TIPS

- Carrots and potatoes are fine for children and can be added to the vegetable mix. If adults are on a stricter low-carb plan, then avoid these.
- To make gravy, pour the juices from the cooked chicken into a saucepan and heat. Add 200 ml fresh cream and bring to the boil, stirring continuously. Cream burns easily, so be aware. For a thicker gravy, add 100 g Philadelphia® cream cheese and 15 ml Worcestershire sauce.

Tarragon chicken with red coleslaw

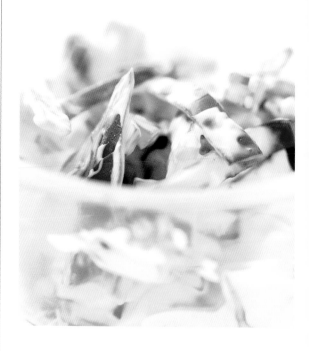

30 ml organic coconut oil or butter
3–4 chicken fillets, cubed
1 onion, chopped
4 cloves garlic, crushed
30 ml dried tarragon
30 ml pink peppercorns
15 ml tomato purée
15 ml Dijon mustard
15 ml ground coriander
10 ml paprika
30 ml chopped fresh parsley
300 ml fresh cream
100 g cashew nuts, chopped (optional)
Salt and pepper
1 red pepper, chopped

Melt the oil or butter and fry the chicken until lightly browned. Add the rest of the ingredients, except the red pepper, and simmer for 10–15 minutes.

Add the red pepper and cook for a further 3 minutes.

Red coleslaw

200 g red cabbage
100 ml mayonnaise
100 ml crème fraîche
5 ml Dijon mustard
Pinch of salt

Finely slice the cabbage into thin strips. Mix the mayonnaise, crème fraîche, mustard and salt together and then mix with the cabbage.

Serve the chicken with red coleslaw and mashed broccoli (see page 122).

 TIP The coleslaw works just as well with any kind of cabbage.

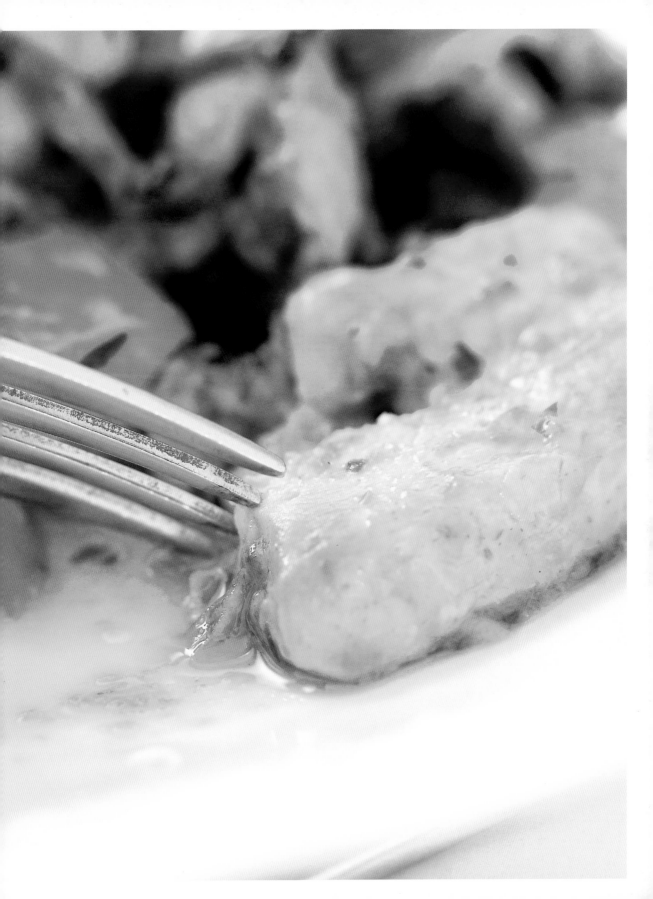

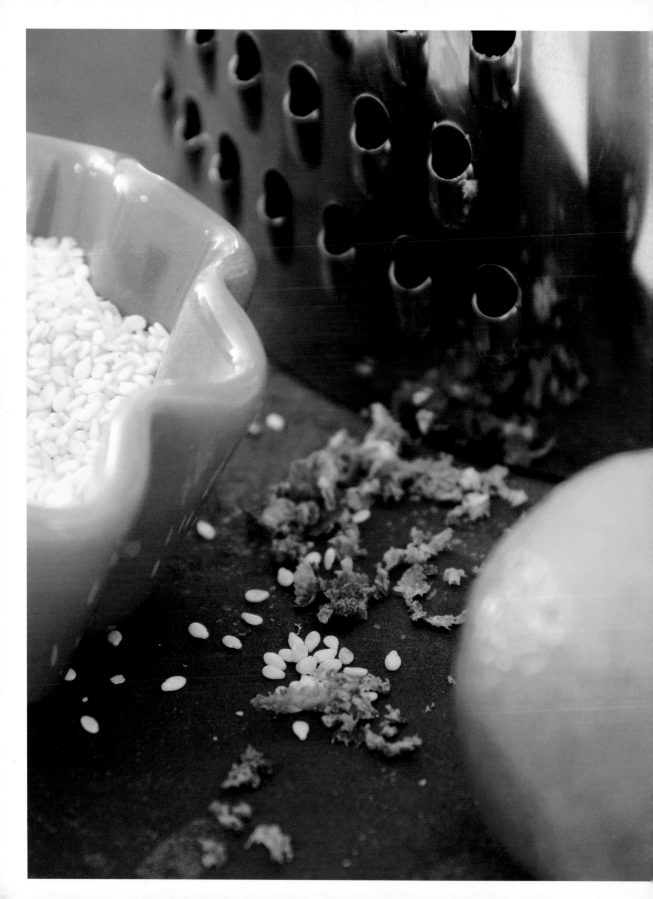

Grilled chicken wings with dipping sauce

30 ml organic coconut oil
20–25 chicken wings or mini drumsticks
Salt and pepper

Preheat the oven to 200 °C. Grease an ovenproof dish with some of the coconut oil.

Season the chicken and place in the prepared dish, evenly spread out. Drizzle with coconut oil and grill in the oven for around 20 minutes.

Marinade

90 ml balsamic vinegar
Juice of 3 limes
Grated zest of 1 lime
30 ml organic coconut oil
15 ml tomato purée
5 ml paprika
100 ml sesame seeds

Mix all the ingredients together in a bowl. Remove the chicken from the oven and pour the marinade over the chicken. Return the chicken to the oven and grill for another 20 minutes, turning the chicken after 10 minutes.

Dipping sauce

200 ml crème fraîche
1 clove garlic, crushed
Salt and pepper
5 ml grated lime zest

Mix all the ingredients together in a bowl.

Serve the chicken with a selection of raw vegetables, such as broccoli, cucumber, sugar snap peas and cauliflower, which are also good dipped in the sauce.

> **TIP**
> You can make a number of variations of the dipping sauce. Crème fraîche can be mixed with curry powder or with fresh herbs such as chives or parsley, or grate some Cheddar cheese and mix with crème fraîche.

Bacon-wrapped chicken with feta filling

100 g feta cheese, cubed
15 ml dried mixed herbs
4 chicken fillets
8 rashers bacon
30 ml organic coconut oil or butter
1 clove garlic, crushed
Salt and pepper
100 ml crème fraîche
300 ml fresh cream

Preheat the oven to 200 °C.

Cut the feta cheese into small pieces and mix with the dried mixed herbs. Divide the mixture in two: one half for the filling and the other half for later.

Slice the chicken fillets in the middle but not all the way through, to make a pocket. Fill the pocket in each fillet with one half of the feta cheese mixture. Wrap each fillet with 2 rashers of bacon, using a toothpick to keep the bacon in place if necessary.

Melt the oil or butter in a frying pan and fry the chicken on both sides until almost cooked right through. Place the chicken in an ovenproof dish.

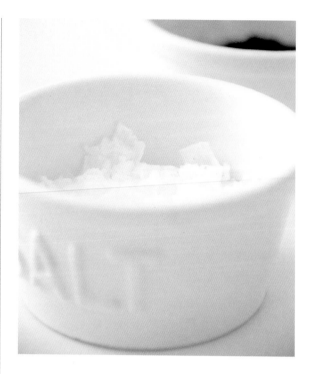

Add the crushed garlic to the remaining feta cheese and herb mixture and add salt and pepper. Melt the feta cheese mixture in the frying pan and stir until the cheese melts. Add the crème fraîche and cream and stir together, and then simmer for a couple of minutes. Pour the sauce over the chicken. Place the chicken in the oven for 15 minutes.

Serve with zucchini tagliatelle (see page 133).

TIP
When buying bacon, avoid those products with added MSG and smoke aroma. Choose bacon that has been smoked the natural way.

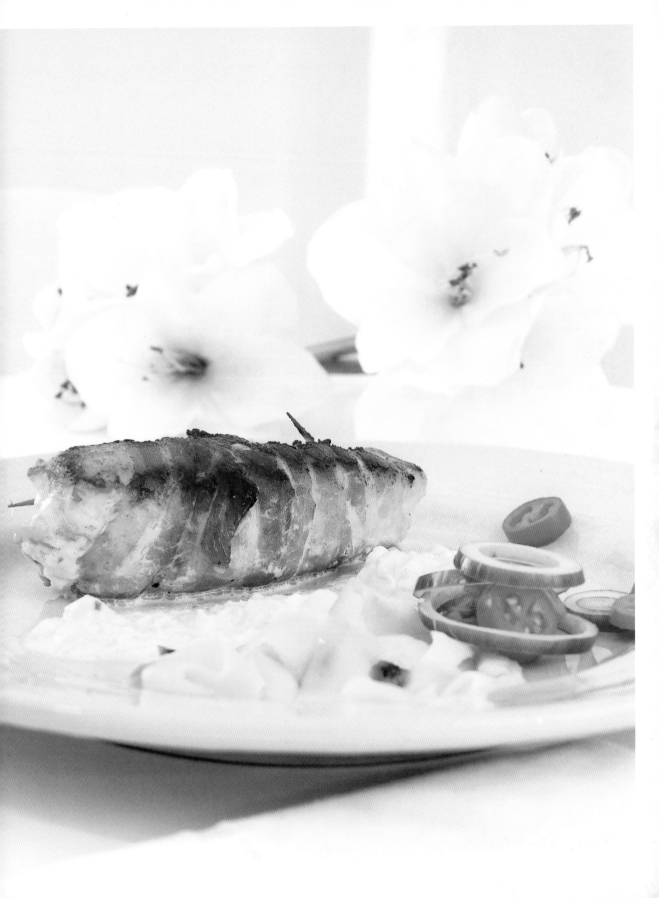

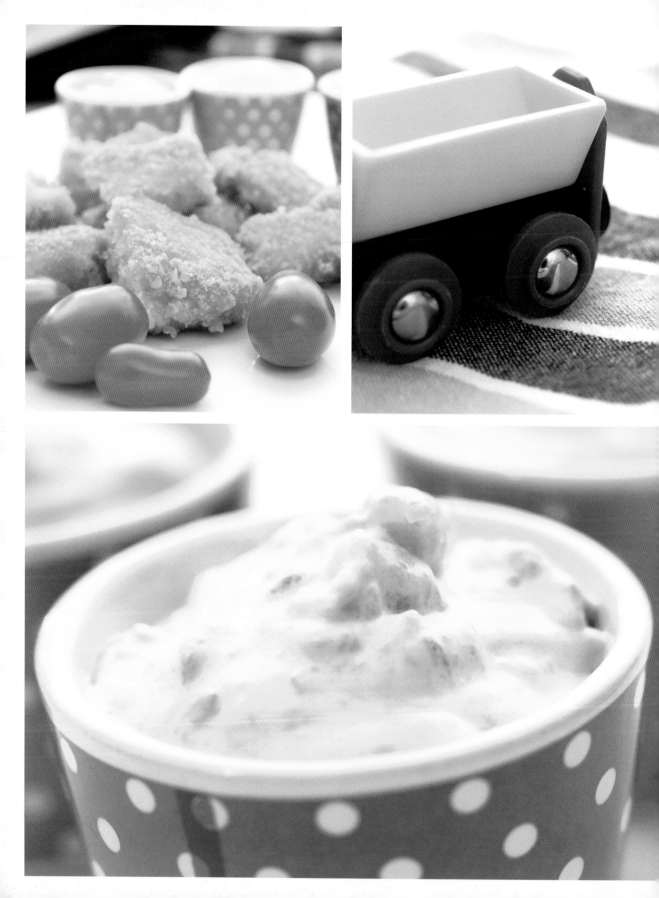

Chicken nuggets with three dipping sauces

4 chicken fillets
150 g pork rind snacks or 150 ml sesame seeds
5 ml garlic powder
1 egg
Salt and pepper
45 ml organic coconut oil

Cut up the chicken into smaller pieces. Process the pork rinds in a blender so that it becomes like a light 'flour'. Add the garlic powder. Beat the egg and season with salt and pepper.

Dip the chicken pieces into the egg and then coat them in the bacon flour (or sesame seeds), making sure each piece of chicken is well covered.

Heat the oil in a frying pan and fry the nuggets until they are golden brown.

Serve with the dipping sauces.

Curry dipping sauce

200 ml crème fraîche
100 ml mayonnaise
15 ml mild curry powder
Salt and pepper

Mix all the ingredients together in a bowl.

Tomato and mustard dipping sauce

15 ml tomato purée
15 ml Dijon mustard
1 clove garlic
150 ml oil (olive or canola)
30 ml mayonnaise

Mix together with a hand blender so that the oil blends with all the other ingredients.

Guacamole

200 ml fresh cream
1 large avocado, mashed
½ onion, finely chopped
15 ml finely chopped red pepper
1 clove garlic, crushed
100 ml crème fraîche

Whip the cream. Stir the mashed avocado, onion, red pepper and garlic into the cream and add the crème fraîche. Stir well.

VARIATION
Add grated Parmesan cheese to the sesame seeds and use this mixture to coat the chicken. Tasty!

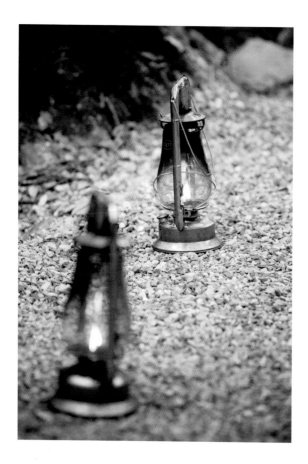

TIP

Use vegetables that grow above the ground because they have fewer carbohydrates than those vegetables that grow below the ground.

Creamy chicken soup with seasonal vegetables

3 chicken fillets
100 g sweet peas
100 g broccoli
100 g cauliflower
100 g baby marrows (courgettes, zucchini)
1 yellow pepper
1 red pepper
1 onion
250 ml chopped fresh parsley
125 ml chopped fresh dill
125 ml snipped chives
Salt and white pepper
500 ml fresh cream
250 ml water (if you find the soup too thick)

Cut up the chicken into smaller pieces. Chop up all the vegetables. Place the chicken, vegetables, herbs and seasoning in a saucepan and add the cream. Bring to the boil, then reduce the heat and simmer for 15 minutes. If necessary, add water for a thinner consistency.

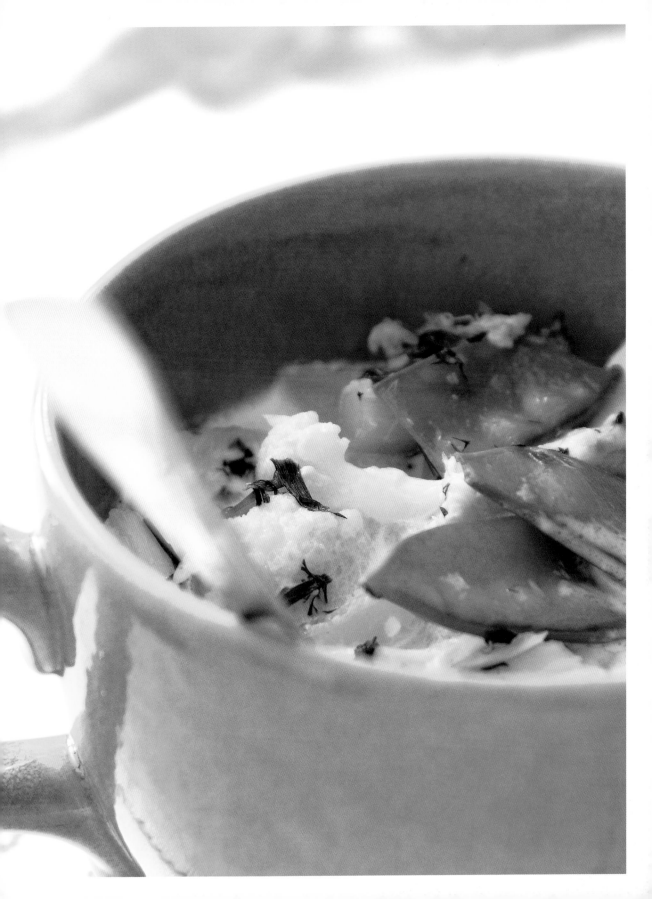

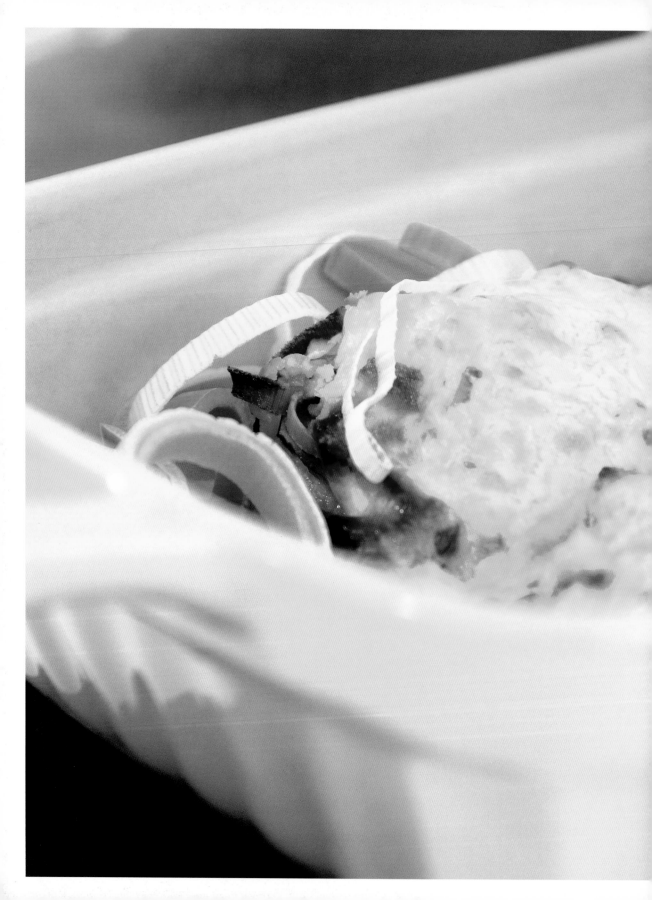

Baked chicken with leek and sun-dried tomato

4 chicken fillets
15 ml organic coconut oil or butter
15 cm-piece leek, chopped
3 cloves garlic, crushed
4–6 sun-dried tomatoes, chopped
500 ml crème fraîche
15 ml Worcestershire sauce
Salt and white pepper
300 ml grated cheese

Preheat the oven to 200 °C.

Brown the chicken in the oil in a frying pan. Place the chicken in an ovenproof dish and bake for 20 minutes.

Mix the leek, garlic, sun-dried tomatoes, crème fraîche, Worcestershire sauce, salt and pepper together in a bowl. Remove the chicken from the oven and pour the sauce over the chicken fillets. Sprinkle the cheese on top and grill in the oven until the cheese has melted and has a golden colour.

Serve with cauliflower rice (see page 129) or with boiled broccoli.

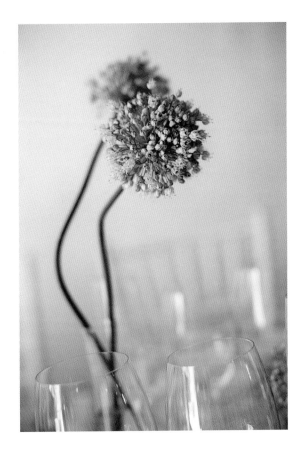

TIP Buy cheese with a high percentage of fat.

Fillet of fish with coconut and horseradish

2 eggs
300 ml coconut flour or almond flour
100 ml sesame seeds
Salt and pepper
3–4 fish fillets
30 ml grated fresh horseradish
30 ml organic coconut oil or butter
A handful of pea shoots

Beat the eggs in a bowl. Mix together the coconut flour and sesame seeds in a separate bowl.

Season the fish fillets and then dip them into the egg. Coat the fish in the flour-seed mixture. Sprinkle a pinch of horseradish on top of the fish.

Heat the oil or butter in a frying pan. Add the rest of the horseradish and fry for a couple of minutes. Place the fish in the pan and fry for 3–5 minutes per side. Remove the fish from the pan and keep warm.

Add the pea shoots to the pan and fry until crisp. Remove from the pan and set aside.

Sauce

15 ml coconut oil or butter
45 ml grated fresh horseradish
200 ml fresh cream
Salt and white pepper
A handful of pea shoots, chopped
30 ml Philadelphia® cream cheese

Using the same frying pan, melt the oil or butter and fry the horseradish for a few seconds. Pour the cream into the pan and add the seasoning and pea shoots. Stir in the cream cheese. Simmer for 7 minutes while stirring.

Decorate the fish with the fried pea shoots. Serve with the sauce and boiled broccoli.

TIP
Philadelphia® cream cheese is great to use in gravy, sauces or stews to give a thicker consistency.

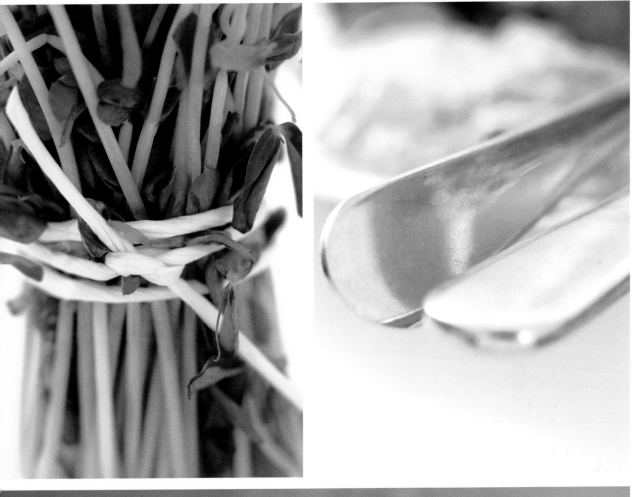
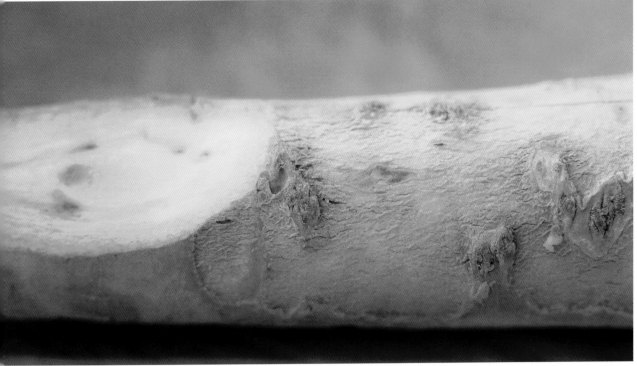

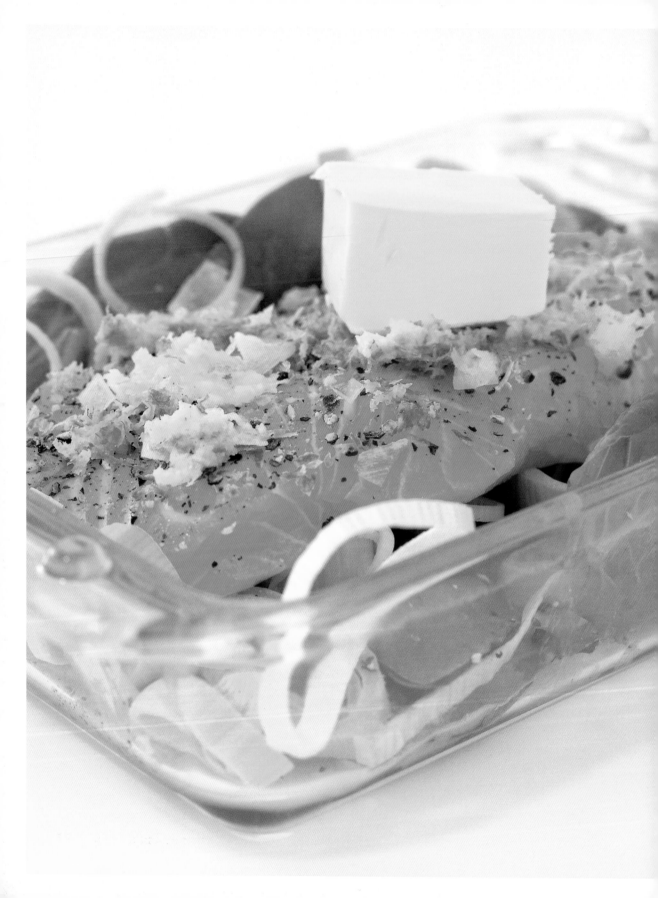

Ginger and garlic-covered salmon with lime butter

60 g organic coconut oil or butter
50 g fresh baby spinach
4 salmon fillets
10 ml sea salt
10 ml pepper
4 cloves garlic, crushed
Grated zest of 2 limes
15 cm-piece leek, sliced
60 ml grated fresh ginger
60 g butter

Preheat the oven to 180 °C. Grease an ovenproof dish with some of the oil or butter.

Place the spinach on the bottom of the prepared dish and spread it out to cover the surface. Lay the salmon fillets on top of the spinach. Season the salmon with salt, pepper and garlic. Sprinkle the lime zest, leek and ginger on top of the salmon. Place 15 ml butter on each piece of salmon and bake for 15–20 minutes.

Lime butter

200 g butter, at room temperature
Grated zest and juice of 1½ limes
Salt and white pepper

Whip the butter using an electric beater and add the lime zest and juice, salt and pepper. Place a sheet of plastic wrap on the kitchen work surface and spoon the butter in a strip in the centre of the plastic. Wrap the plastic around the butter and seal the ends. Shape the butter into a long sausage shape and refrigerate.

Just before serving, cut the butter into 1 cm-thick slices. Serve the butter with the salmon. Mashed cauliflower (see page 122) works well with this dish.

TIP

Fresh baby spinach can be eaten raw or cooked. It is a great source of vitamins A, C and K, manganese and folic acid. Important minerals such as magnesium and potassium are also found in spinach, as is vitamin B_5, iron, phosphorus, copper, zinc and fibre. Children under the age of one should not eat spinach.

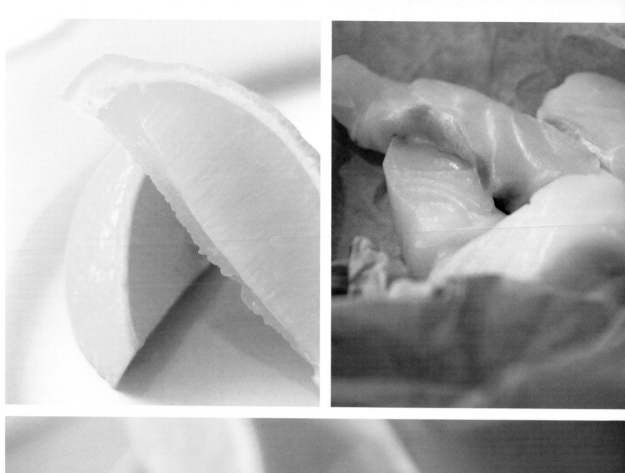

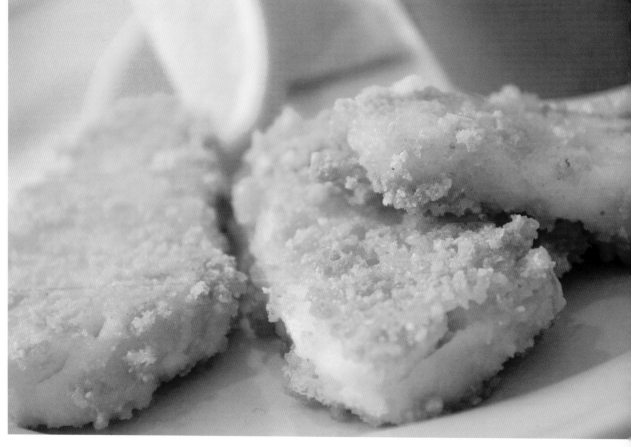

Fish fingers with a cold herb sauce

2 eggs
150 g pork rind snacks
Salt
100 g organic coconut oil or butter
4 fish fillets

Beat the eggs in a bowl. Process the pork rinds in a blender so that it becomes like a light 'flour'. Add salt.

Melt the oil or butter in a frying pan. Cut the fish into fingers. Dip each piece into egg, and then cover the fish with the pork rind 'flour'. Fry the fish for a few minutes on each side.

TIPS
- This recipe works well with whole fillets of fish too.
- Add your favourite spices to the pork flour for extra flavour.

Herb sauce

200 ml crème fraîche
100 ml mayonnaise
125 ml chopped fresh herbs (parsley, dill, chives)
Salt and pepper
15 ml vinegar

Mix all the ingredients together.

Serve as a cold dipping sauce with the fish fingers, mashed broccoli (see page 122) and tomatoes.

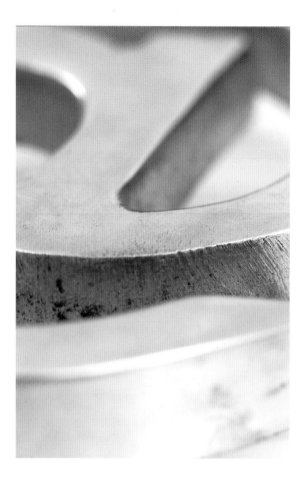

Fish casserole with crispy bacon bits

4 fish fillets
1 onion, chopped
300 ml fresh cream
200 ml crème fraîche
100 g Philadelphia® cream cheese
30 ml tomato purée
Salt and white pepper
300 ml grated cheese
15 ml organic coconut oil or butter
150 g bacon, diced
20 Brussels sprouts
30 ml butter

Preheat the oven to 200 °C. Grease an ovenproof dish.

Cut the fish into bite-sized chunks and place in the prepared dish. Scatter the onion over the fish.

Mix the cream, crème fraîche, cream cheese, tomato purée, salt and pepper together in a bowl. Pour the sauce over the fish and bake for 20 minutes.

Remove the dish from the oven and sprinkle the grated cheese on top, covering the fish. Return to the oven until the cheese becomes golden in colour.

Heat the oil or butter in a frying pan and fry the bacon until crisp. Sprinkle the bacon over the casserole dish.

Cook the Brussels sprouts in boiling water for 5–8 minutes. Drain the water, add the butter and allow to melt. Make sure all the Brussels sprouts are covered and glazed with butter. Serve with the fish casserole.

TIP
Not all children enjoy Brussels sprouts. Alternatively, boil a potato and mash with butter or serve the casserole with mashed avocado.

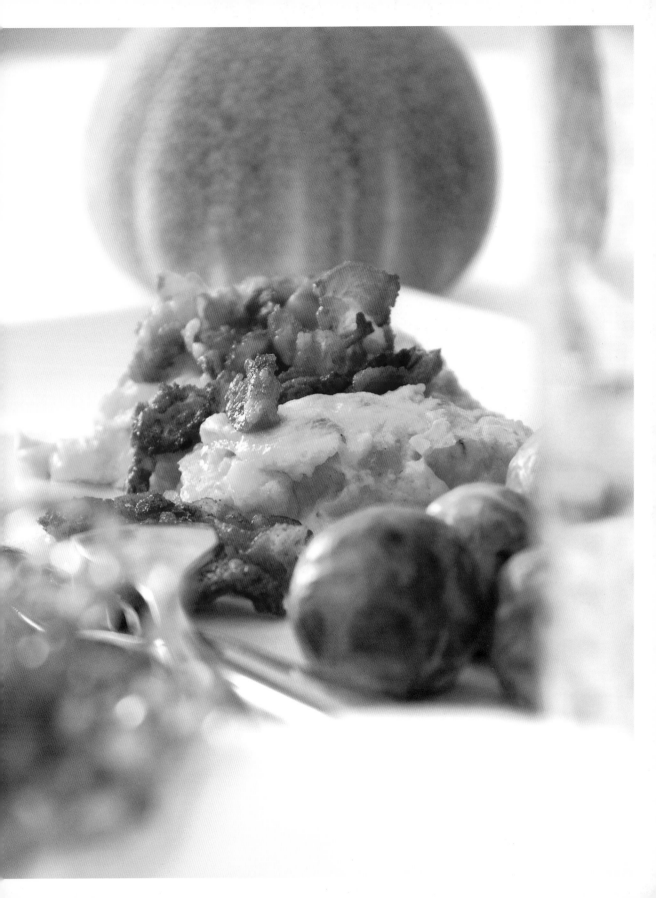

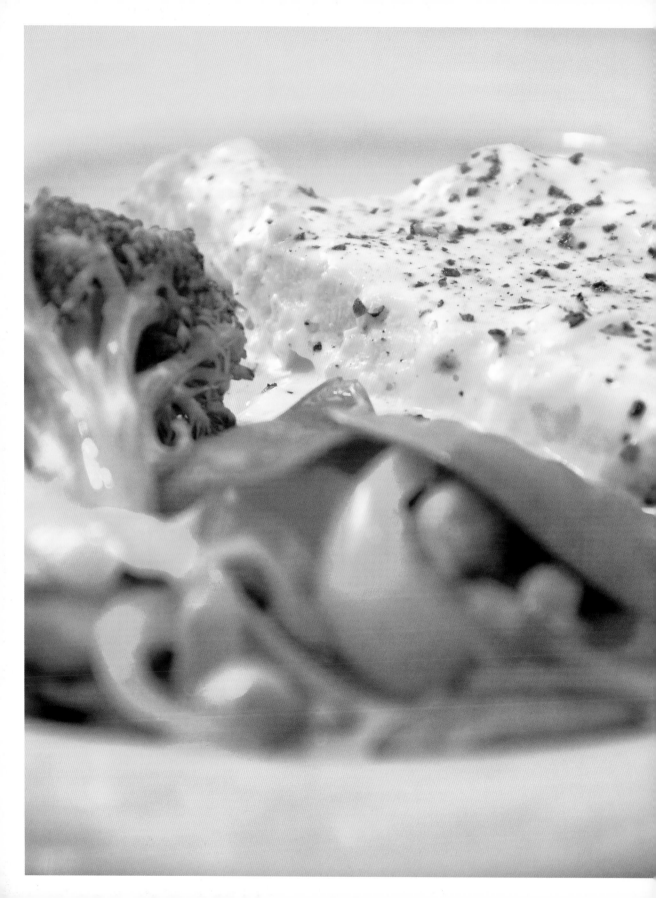

Salmon with creamy cheese sauce and butter-fried vegetable stir-fry

500 ml crème fraîche
200 ml fresh cream
Salt and pepper
Pinch of cayenne pepper
2 cloves garlic
30 ml dry white wine (optional)
4 salmon fillets
30 ml butter
300 ml grated cheese (Parmesan or Cheddar works well)

Preheat the oven to 180 °C. Grease an ovenproof dish.

Mix the crème fraîche, cream, seasoning, cayenne pepper, garlic and wine together in a saucepan over medium heat and simmer for around 3 minutes.

Place the salmon fillets in the prepared dish. Place a knob of butter on each piece of salmon. Cover the salmon with the grated cheese and pour the sauce over the top. Bake for 30 minutes.

Vegetable stir-fry

100 g butter
1 yellow pepper
4 broccoli florets
8 sugar snap peas
10 cm-piece leek
4 mushrooms, quartered
Salt and pepper

Melt the butter in a wok or pan. Chop the vegetables into chunks and fry them in the butter. The vegetables should still be crisp, so only fry for a short time, say 5–8 minutes.

Serve the vegetables with the fish.

TIP
I avoid using stock when making food. If you do use stock or broth, make sure you read the ingredients and avoid MSG. Aim for raw spices that are free from additives.

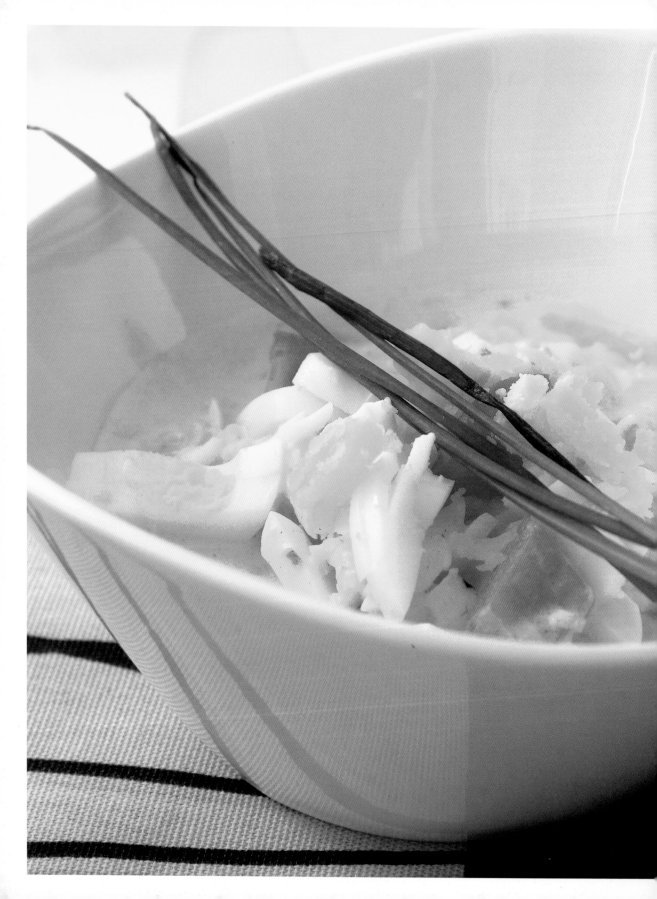

Fish stew

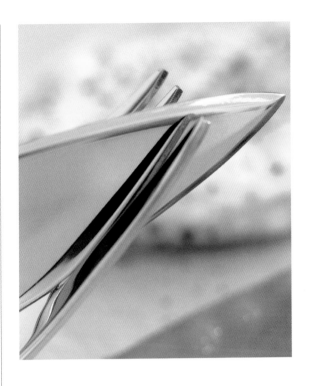

30 ml organic coconut oil or butter
400 g fish of choice
500 ml fresh cream
30 ml Dijon mustard
Salt and pepper
Juice of 1 lemon
3 hard-boiled eggs, finely chopped
3 tomatoes, finely chopped

Melt the oil or butter in a saucepan. Cut the fish into bite-sized pieces and fry in the oil for a few minutes. Add the cream and mustard, salt, pepper and lemon juice. Simmer for 15 minutes.

Mix the eggs and tomatoes together and add to the fish stew just before serving. Don't let it boil.

Serve with boiled asparagus or broccoli.

TIP You can add a few knobs of butter to the vegetables to increase the fat content.

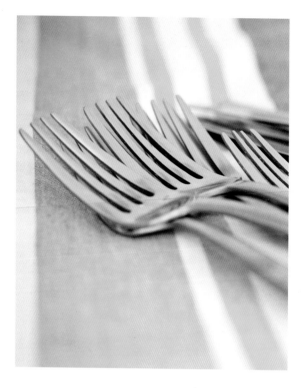

Cabbage 'spaghetti' with tuna

2 tins tuna in water, drained
200 ml fresh cream
300 ml crème fraîche
100 g Philadelphia® cream cheese
15 ml curry powder
Juice of 1 lemon
100 ml chopped fresh parsley
Salt and white pepper
250 g cabbage

Spoon the tuna into a saucepan. Add the cream, crème fraîche, cream cheese and curry powder. Add the lemon juice and parsley. Bring to the boil and simmer for 5 minutes. Season to taste.

Shred the cabbage and boil in salted water for around 5 minutes.

Spoon the cabbage onto plates and pour the tuna sauce over the top.

TIP

Although I eat strictly LCHF, I choose tuna in water. This is due to the fact that tuna is often in sunflower oil, which contains a huge amount of omega-6. We already take in enough omega-6, and too much of it isn't good for you.

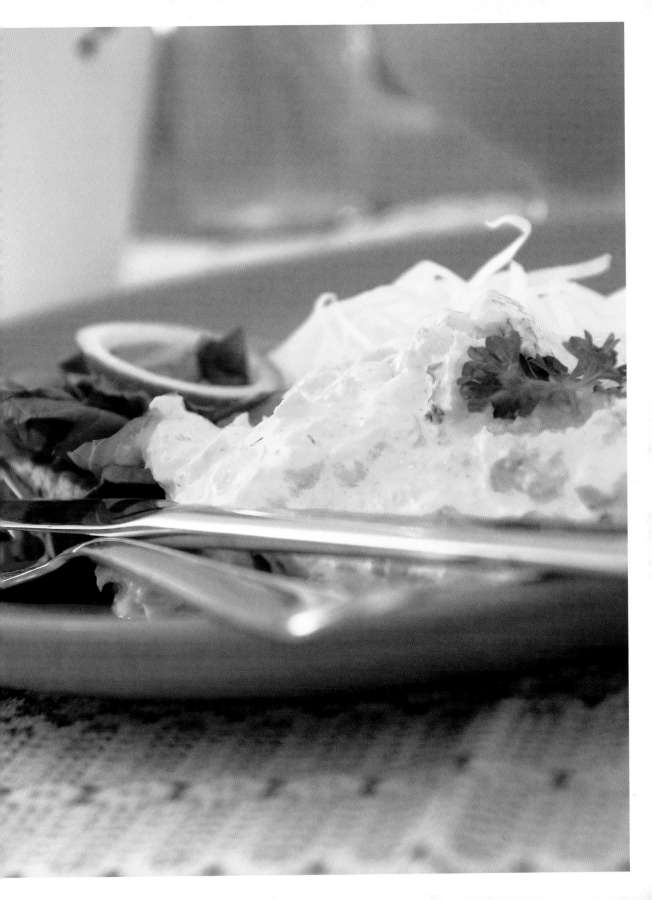

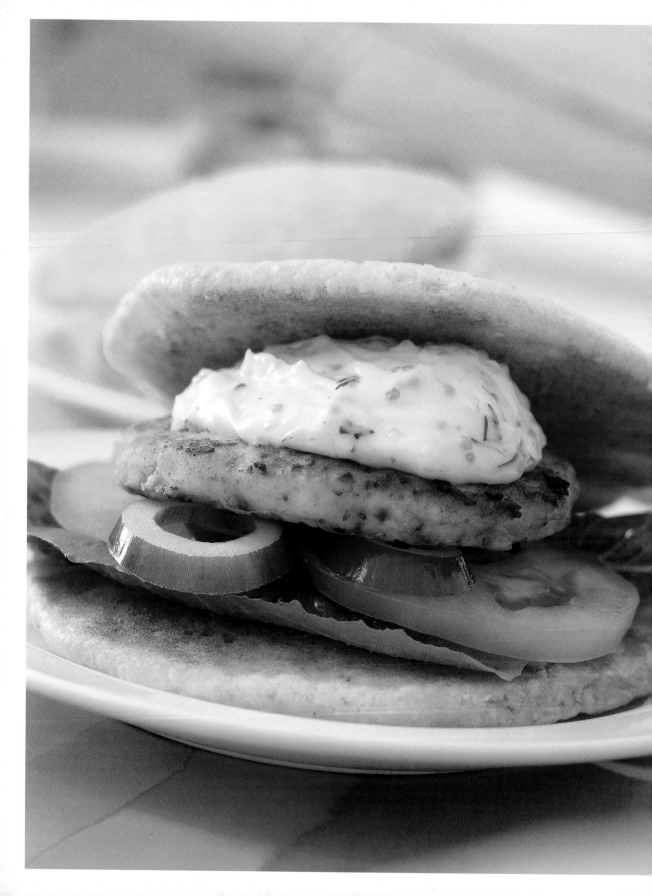

Salmon burger with a creamy dressing

400 g salmon fillets
100 g white fish
½ onion, chopped
1 clove garlic, crushed
Grated zest and juice of 1 lemon
2 eggs, beaten
Salt and pepper
50 g organic coconut oil or butter for frying

Cut the fish into smaller pieces and make sure there are no bones. Place the fish, onion, garlic and lemon zest and juice in a food processor and blend until it forms a coarse mixture. Stir in the eggs and salt and pepper. Form the mixture into burger patties.

Melt the oil or butter in a frying pan and fry the burgers over medium heat for around 8 minutes on each side, turning regularly.

Creamy dressing

100 ml mayonnaise
200 ml crème fraîche
15 ml caviar (optional)
15 ml chopped fresh dill
Juice of ½ lemon
Salt and pepper

Mix all the ingredients together in a bowl and season to taste. Refrigerate until needed.

Serve the salmon burgers with LCHF bread rolls (see right), sliced tomatoes, lettuce and creamy dressing.

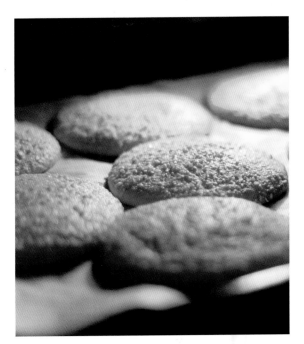

LCHF bread rolls

200 ml sesame seeds, plus extra for sprinkling
100 ml coconut flour (available from health stores, alternatively use almond flour)
15 ml psyllium husk (available from health stores)
Salt
10 ml baking powder
2 eggs
200 ml fresh cream
100 ml grated cheese

Preheat the oven to 200 °C. Line a baking tray with baking paper.

Blend the sesame seeds in a food processor or with a hand blender until it forms 'flour'. Add the coconut flour, psyllium husk, salt and baking powder.

Mix the eggs and cream together and add the cheese. Add the egg mixture to the flour mixture and mix well. Place about 30 ml of the mixture in heaps on the prepared tray. Sprinkle some sesame seeds on top of each bun and bake for 15 minutes.

TIPS
- I use one roll on the top and one at the bottom of the burger, as they are very dense and filling.
- You can also eat these bread rolls at breakfast time.

Butter-fried salmon with glazed chive tomatoes and coriander cream sauce

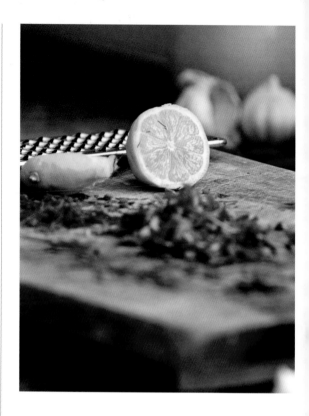

Butter-fried salmon

100 g butter
100 ml snipped garlic chives or chives
100 ml chopped fresh coriander
50 ml chopped fresh dill
800 g salmon fillets
Grated zest of ½ lemon

Coriander cream sauce

300 ml crème fraîche
150 ml finely chopped fresh coriander
Salt and pepper
Juice of ½ lemon

Glazed chive tomatoes

50 g butter
250 g cocktail tomatoes
30 ml snipped garlic chives or chives

TIP

You can use other herbs in the cold sauce, such as parsley, dill or even crushed garlic, if you prefer.

Butter-fried salmon

Heat the butter in a saucepan and add half the chives, coriander and dill. Place the salmon fillets in the pan and sprinkle with the rest of the herbs and the lemon zest. Fry the fish over low heat for around 8 minutes. Carefully turn over and fry the other side for another 8 minutes. Keep warm.

Coriander cream sauce

Mix all the ingredients together and refrigerate.

Glazed chive tomatoes

Melt the butter in a saucepan and add the tomatoes. Stir in the chives and fry for a couple of minutes until glazed.

Place the fish on a serving platter and spoon the tomatoes around it. Serve with the cold sauce.

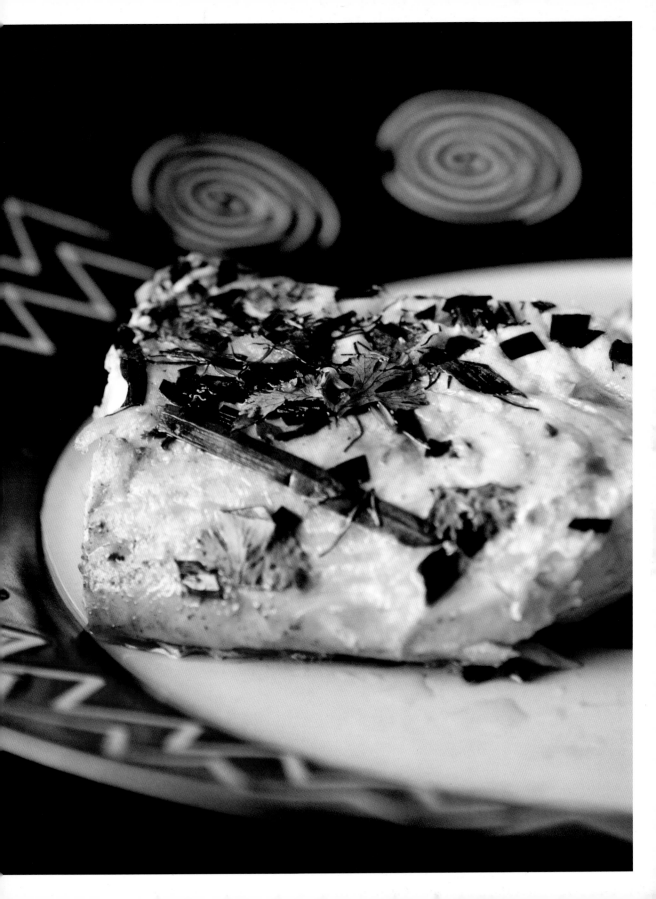

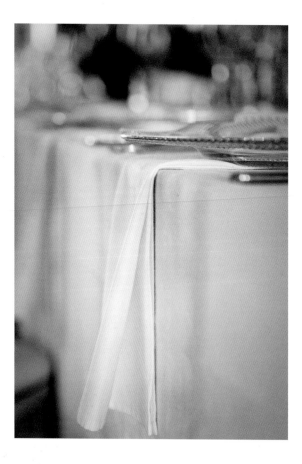

Fish stew with dill and prawns

100 g organic coconut oil or butter
1 onion, chopped
4–8 mushrooms, sliced
10 cm baby marrow (courgette, zucchini),
    chopped
1 yellow pepper, chopped
4 broccoli florets
Grated zest and juice of 1 lemon
Salt and pepper
200 ml fresh cream
200 ml crème fraîche
200 g Philadelphia® cream cheese
15 ml tomato purée
15 ml Dijon mustard
30 ml chopped fresh dill
400 g fish of choice, cut into bite-sized pieces
100 g peeled cooked prawns

Melt the oil or butter in a saucepan and fry the onion
and the mushrooms. Add the baby marrow, yellow
pepper and broccoli and fry together for a few minutes.
Stir in the lemon zest and juice.

Add the seasoning, cream, crème fraîche, cream
cheese, tomato purée, mustard and dill, and stir. Add
the fish to the stew and simmer until the fish is cooked,
around 10 minutes.

Remove from the heat and add the prawns. Serve the
stew as is or with boiled asparagus.

TIP Use whichever vegetables are in
season and that your family enjoys.

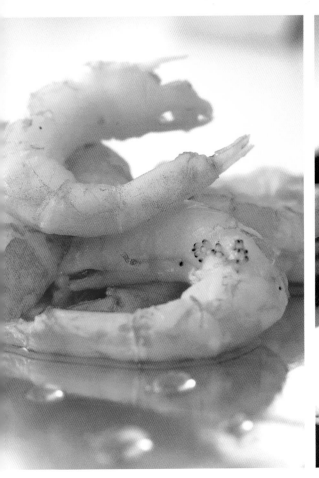

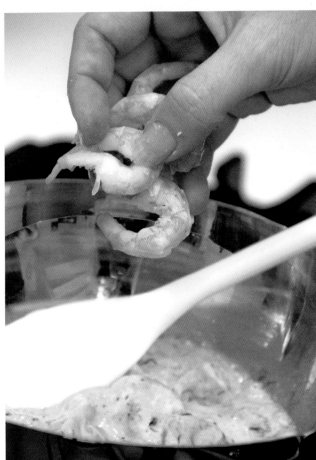

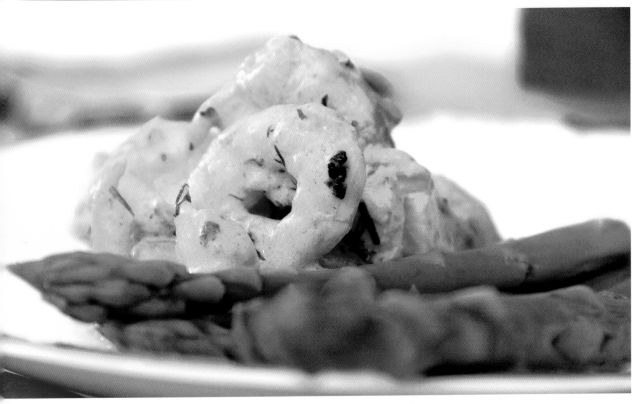

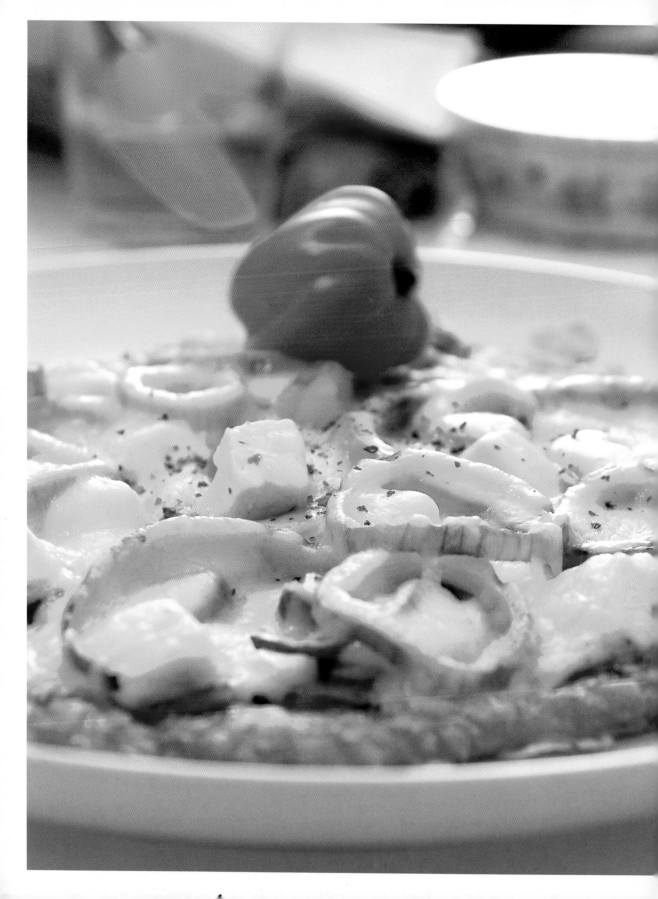

Pizza

1 serving

2 eggs
200 ml grated cheese (use any hard cheese like
Cheddar or Gouda)
25 ml tomato purée

Topping

Selection of your favourite topping ingredients
200 ml grated cheese

Preheat the oven to 200 °C.

Whisk the eggs and add the grated cheese. Spread the mixture in a circle on a baking sheet on a baking tray. Bake the pizza base for around 10 minutes. Remove from the oven when it is crisp and golden brown.

Spread the tomato purée over the pizza base and add your favourite topping. Sprinkle over the grated cheese and place in the oven for around 10 minutes until the cheese has melted.

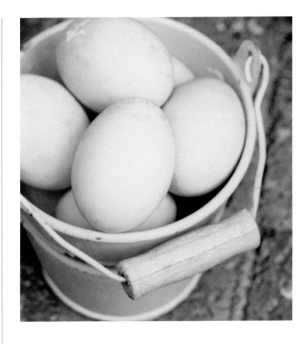

TIPS
- If you wish to make a family-sized pizza, then double or quadruple the quantities for the base.
- Toppings can include ham, tomato, onion, mushrooms, Brie cheese, olives, feta cheese, peppers, etc.

Risotto with cauliflower 'rice'

50 g butter
1 onion, chopped
2 cloves garlic, crushed
200 ml white wine
500 ml cauliflower rice (see page 129)
500 ml fresh cream
1 egg yolk

Melt the butter in a frying pan and sauté the onion and garlic. Add the wine and bring to the boil. Reduce the heat and simmer for 5 minutes. Add the cauliflower rice. Pour in half the cream and simmer for another 8–10 minutes until the cream thickens. If it becomes too dry, add more cream. The risotto should be creamy. Remove from the heat and stir in the egg yolk.

> **TIP**
> The secrets of a good risotto are not to use more than two main ingredients and to find two main ingredients that taste good together.

VARIATIONS TO ADD TO THE RISOTTO

Prawns and asparagus

6 asparagus spears, boiled
300 g peeled cooked prawns

Add the asparagus to the risotto at the same time as you add the cream. Only add the prawns right at the end.

Bacon and mushroom

50 g organic coconut oil or butter
150 g bacon, diced
100 g mushrooms, sliced

Melt half the oil or butter in a frying pan and fry the bacon until cooked to your liking. Remove from the pan and set aside. Melt the rest of the oil in the pan and fry the mushrooms until crisp. Mix the bacon and mushrooms into the risotto when you add the cream.

Chicken and broccoli

50 g organic coconut oil or butter
3–4 chicken fillets, thinly sliced
Salt and pepper
Pinch of paprika
½ head broccoli, broken into small florets

Melt the oil or butter in a frying pan and fry the chicken. Add the seasoning and paprika. Add the broccoli when the chicken has a golden colour and fry together for a few minutes. Remove from the heat. Add the chicken and broccoli mix to the simmering risotto.

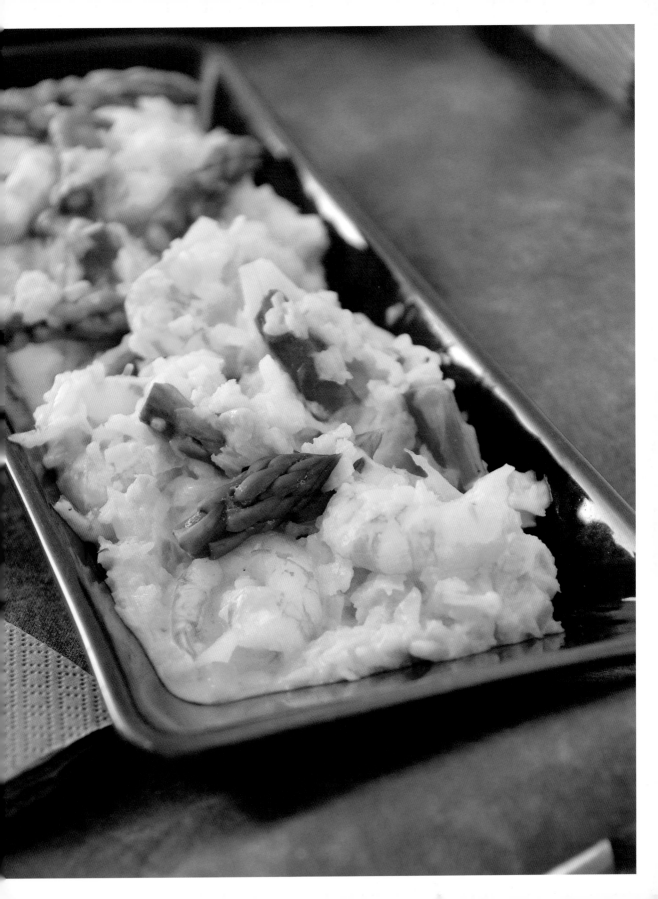

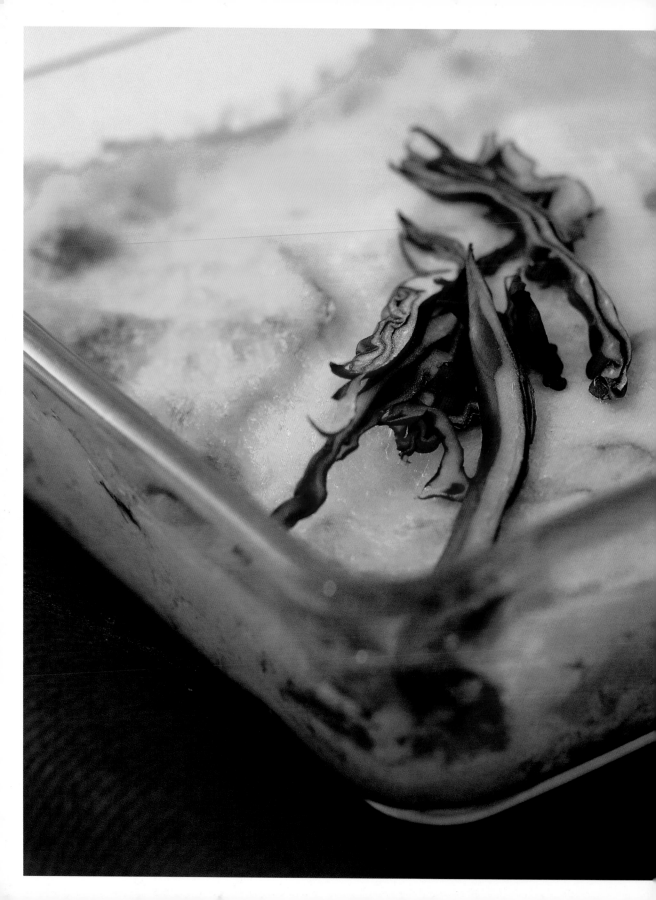

Quick and simple oven bake

6 hard-boiled eggs, sliced
150 g ham or sausage (at least 80% meat), diced
100 g mushrooms, sliced
200 ml mayonnaise
200 ml crème fraîche
100 ml Dijon mustard
Salt and white pepper
300 ml grated cheese

Preheat the oven to 200 °C.

Arrange the egg slices on the bottom of a casserole dish. Layer the ham or sausage on top of the eggs and then top with sliced mushrooms.

Mix the mayonnaise, crème fraîche, mustard, salt and pepper together and pour into the casserole dish, covering the egg and meat mixture. Sprinkle grated cheese over the top and bake for 15–20 minutes.

Serve with a salad.

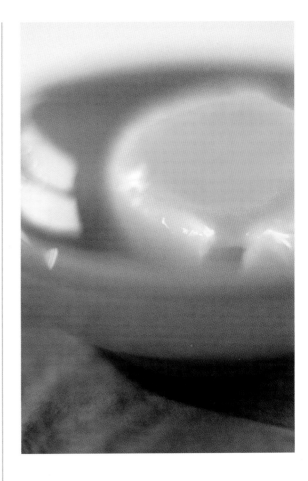

TIP This very easy dish is perfect for a brunch or light supper.

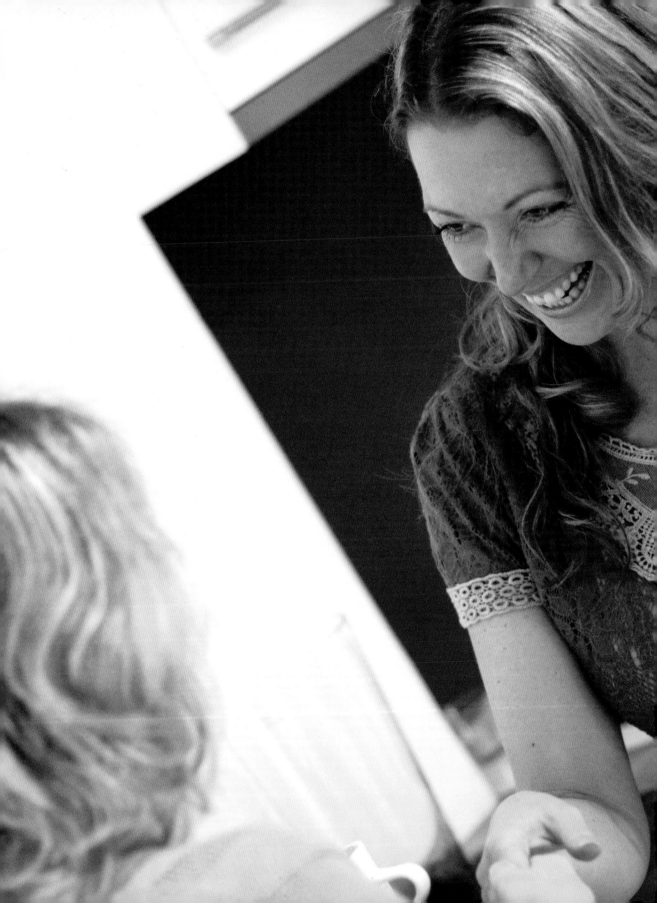

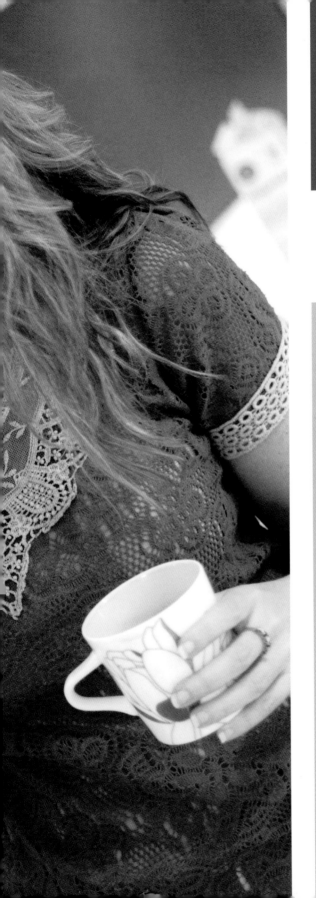

Sides and sauces

The low-carb eating plan focuses primarily on protein and fat. Accompaniments and extras therefore add variation, vitamins, antioxidants, colour and flavour to your meals.

In the beginning it might feel strange not to eat potatoes, rice or pasta with your meal, but you will soon get used to the idea and will find new alternatives to carbs, to make your food enjoyable but still within the LCHF eating plan.

Here are a few of my family's favourite extras.

Mashed broccoli or cauliflower

4 servings

200 ml fresh cream
2 heads broccoli or 1 head cauliflower, broken
   into florets
Salt and pepper
1 clove garlic, crushed (optional)
15 ml butter

Pour the cream into a saucepan and add the broccoli or cauliflower. Bring to the boil, but keep an eye on it as cream boils over easily. Reduce the heat and simmer for 15 minutes.

Add the seasoning and garlic and mix with a hand blender until smooth. Add the butter and stir until the butter has melted.

VARIATION
Cook the broccoli or cauliflower in boiling water. Drain and add 150 g butter, seasoning and garlic. Mix with a hand blender until smooth.

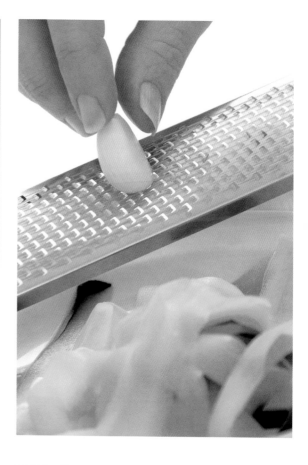

TIP You can prepare either broccoli or cauliflower, or you can make a mix of both, which is very popular with my family.

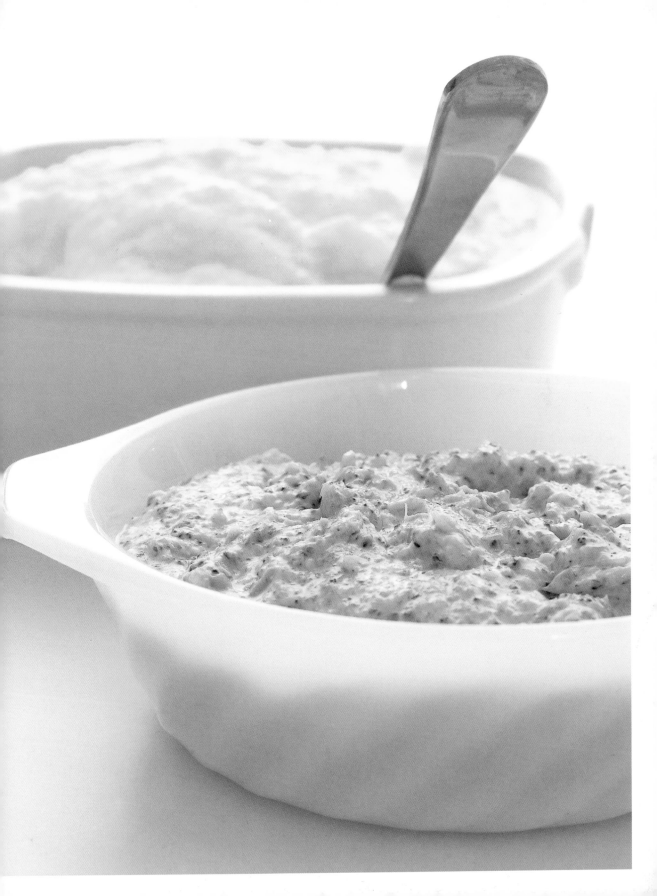

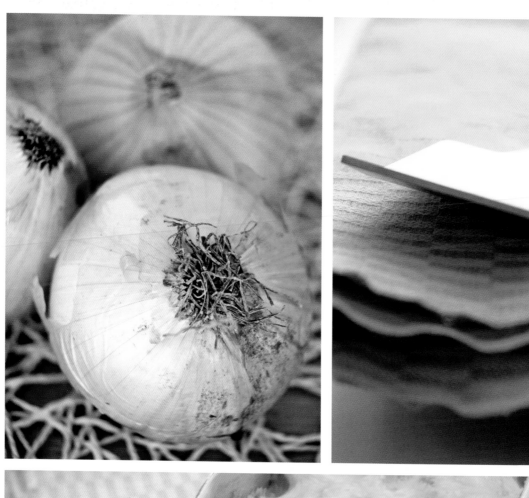
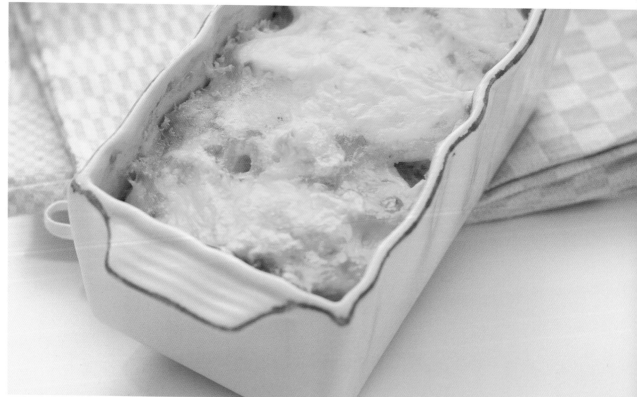

Fennel gratin

4 servings

300 ml crème fraîche
300 ml fresh cream
200 g Philadelphia® cream cheese
3–5 cloves garlic, crushed
Salt and pepper
400 g fennel, sliced
2 onions, sliced into rings
300 ml grated cheese (Cheddar works well)

Preheat the oven to 150 °C.

Mix the crème fraîche, cream, cream cheese, garlic, salt and pepper together in a bowl.

Arrange a layer of fennel and onions in an ovenproof dish and pour over the cream mixture. Bake in the oven for 45 minutes, or until the fennel is soft. Remove from the oven and sprinkle the cheese over the top. Bake for another 10 minutes until the cheese is melted and golden in colour.

Serve with steak, cold meats or chicken.

TIP You can also prepare this dish with other vegetables that grow above ground, such as broccoli and cauliflower.

Broccoli mix

4 servings

1 head broccoli, broken into florets
30 ml crème fraîche
30 ml mayonnaise
Salt and pepper
30 ml chopped fresh parsley
15 ml snipped chives
15 ml chopped fresh coriander
100 ml grated cheese

Cook the broccoli in boiling water for a few minutes and then drain. Place the rest of the ingredients in a bowl and add the broccoli to this. Mix together.

Serve warm or cold as a side dish or salad. Lovely with a barbecue.

TIP Side dishes and mixes are easy to prepare. Use your imagination and experiment with different low-carb ingredients.

Guacamole

4 servings

3 avocados, peeled and depipped
2 cloves garlic, crushed
1–2 drops Tabasco®
Pinch of cayenne pepper
200 ml crème fraîche
Juice of ½ lime
½ red pepper, finely chopped
Salt and pepper

Mash all the ingredients together using a fork. For a smooth consistency, use a blender.

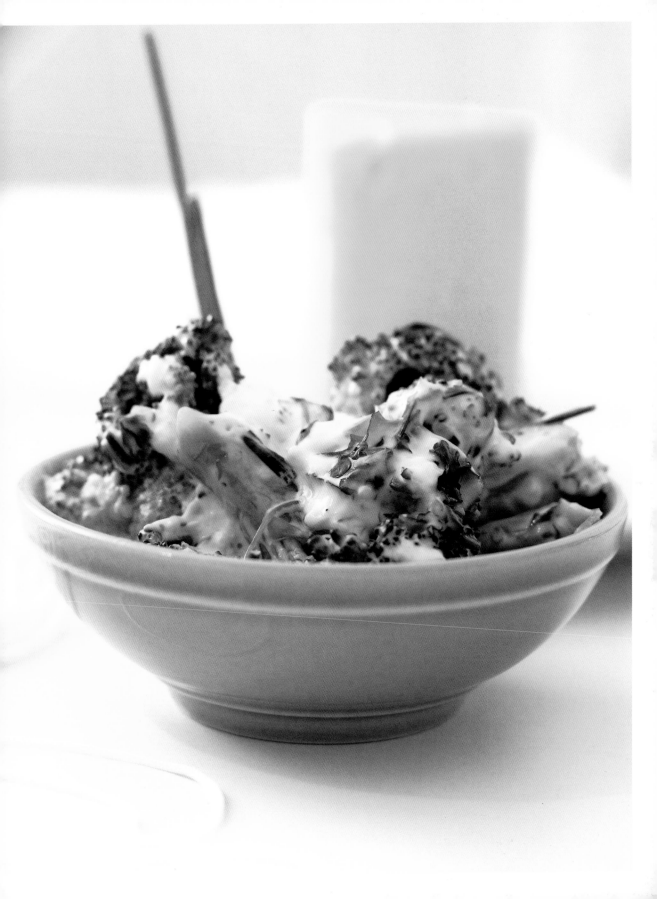

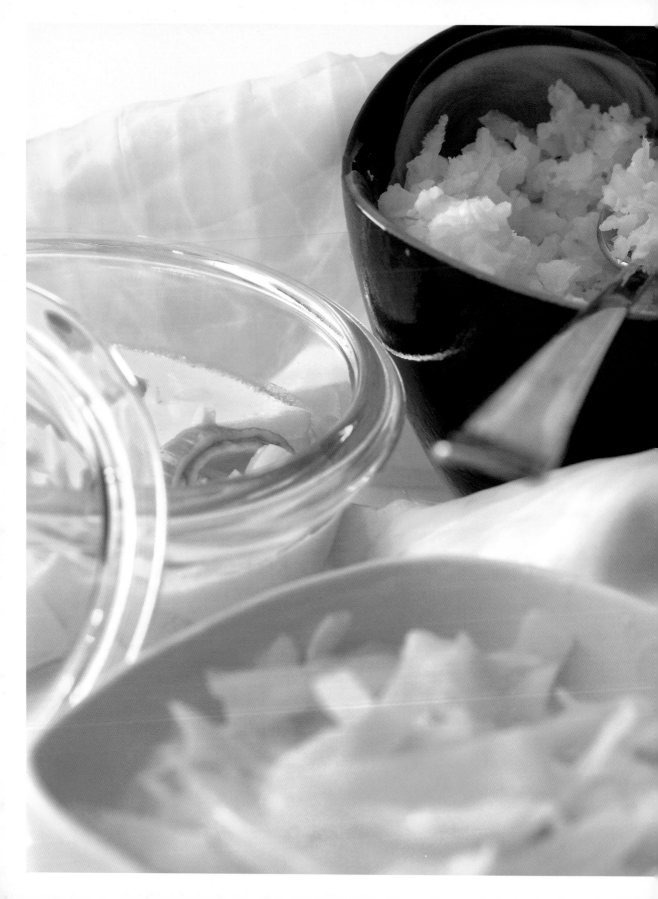

Creamy leek and baby marrow

4 servings

30 ml butter
1 leek, thinly sliced
**10 baby marrows (courgettes, zucchini), thinly
    sliced**
200 ml fresh cream
Pinch of cayenne pepper
Salt

Melt the butter in a saucepan and fry the leek and baby marrow for a few minutes. Pour in the cream and add the cayenne pepper and salt. Bring to the boil and then reduce the heat and simmer until it thickens.

Serve with meat, fish or chicken dishes.

> **TIP**
> We are so used to having rice, pasta, potatoes or fries with our meals, but we just need to re-think and find new and healthy alternatives.

Creamy cabbage

4 servings

½ medium cabbage
200 ml fresh cream
Pinch of white pepper
Salt
15 ml butter
1 egg yolk

Grate the cabbage with a cheese grater and place in a saucepan. Add the cream and bring to the boil. Reduce the heat and simmer for 10–15 minutes. Add the seasoning and remove from the heat. Stir in the butter and egg yolk.

Serve with chicken or meat dishes.

Cauliflower rice

4 servings

1 head cauliflower
1 litre water
Salt
50 g butter

Grate the cauliflower on the coarse side of a cheese grater. Bring the water and salt to the boil in a saucepan. Add the cauliflower to the boiling water and boil for 3 minutes. Drain the cauliflower in a colander.

Transfer the cauliflower rice to a serving bowl and add the butter on top so that it melts into the rice.

Serve with stews.

Luxurious salad

Romaine or cos lettuce
Avocado
Baby marrows (courgettes, zucchini)
Mushrooms
Spring onions
Broccoli
Green pepper
Green asparagus
Baby spinach
Leek
Blueberries (optional)

All the ingredients should be fresh and raw, except the asparagus, which you can boil slightly. Cut up all the ingredients, except the blueberries, and arrange on a platter or mix in a salad bowl. Scatter the blueberries over the top.

TIP Kids most often enjoy salad ingredients when they are all served separately. This way they can then pick and choose what they like.

Tomato salad
4 servings

3 tomatoes, thinly sliced
1 red onion, thinly sliced into rings
30 ml olive oil
10 ml tarragon vinegar or other vinegar
Salt and white pepper
15 ml chopped fresh tarragon or parsley

Layer the slices of tomatoes and onion in a shallow dish. Mix the remaining ingredients together and pour over the salad.

TIP Children often prefer salads or vegetables without dressing. In this case, serve the dressing on the side.

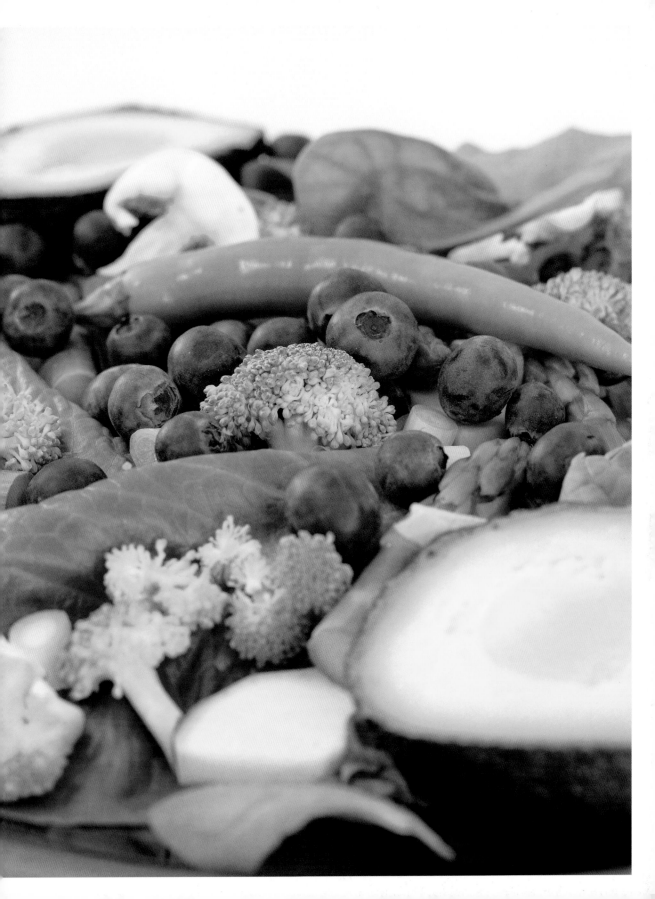

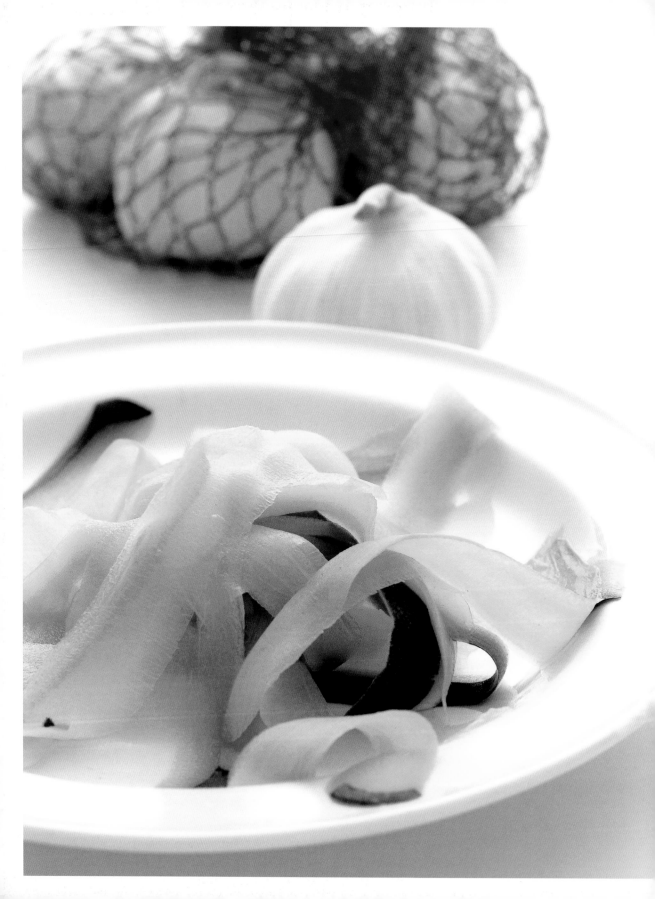

Zucchini 'tagliatelle'

4 servings

10 baby marrows (courgettes, zucchini)
30 ml organic coconut oil or butter
1–2 cloves garlic, crushed

Using a cheese slicer or potato peeler, slice the baby marrow into long strips.

Melt the oil or butter in a frying pan over medium heat. Add the garlic and baby marrow strips. Carefully mix together and fry for a couple of minutes. Remove from the heat before it gets too soft.

Serve with meat, chicken or fish dishes or with a filling sauce in place of pasta.

Monique's lovely dipping sauce

Makes around 350 ml

100 ml olive oil or avocado oil
100 ml white vinegar
30 ml Dijon mustard
15 ml tomato purée
100 ml mayonnaise

Blend all the ingredients together with an electric hand blender so that the oil blends in with the other ingredients.

Serve with prawns, raw vegetables or other 'finger foods'.

TIP The dipping sauce can also be used as a dressing for burgers, fish, prawns or chicken nuggets.

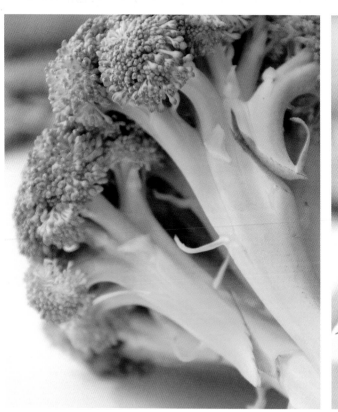
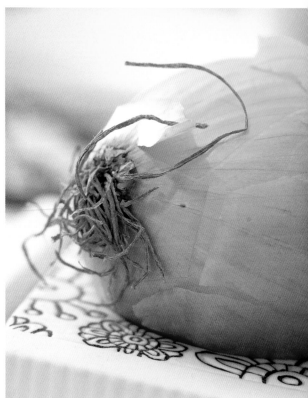
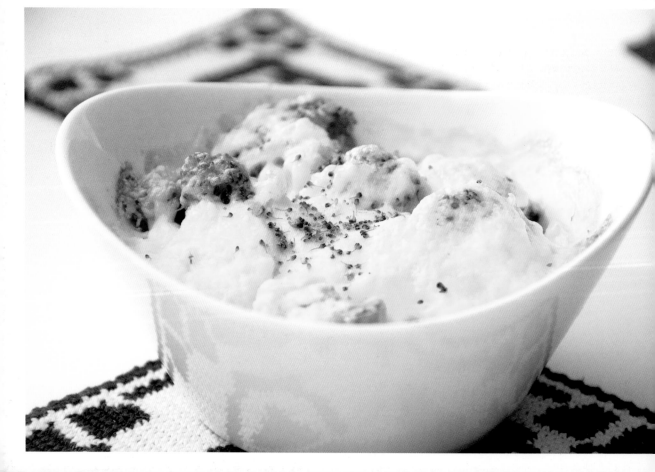

Baked broccoli

4 servings

1 head broccoli, broken into florets
1 onion, sliced into rings
100 g Philadelphia® cream cheese
200 ml crème fraîche
100 ml fresh cream
2 cloves garlic, crushed
Salt and white pepper
200 ml grated cheese

Preheat the oven to 180 °C.

Layer the broccoli florets and onion rings in an ovenproof dish.

Mix the cream cheese, crème fraîche, cream, garlic and seasoning together in a bowl. Pour the mixture over the broccoli and onion and use a fork to help the sauce run in-between the vegetables. Bake for 30–40 minutes.

Remove the dish from the oven and sprinkle the grated cheese over the top. Set the oven to grill and return the dish to the oven until the cheese is golden brown.

TIP You can prepare this dish with just about any vegetable. The cream cheese makes it creamy and thick.

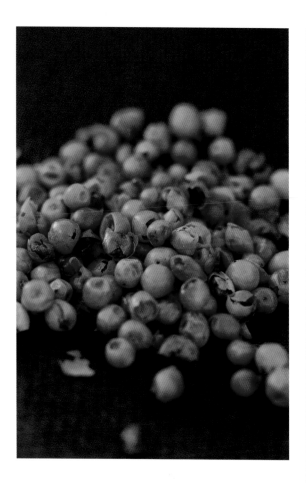

Pepper sauce
4 servings

**45 ml black peppercorns (or a mix of black,
white and pink peppercorns)**
50 g organic coconut oil or butter
10 cm-piece leek, finely chopped
200 ml fresh cream
Salt
30 ml crème fraîche

Coarsely chop the peppercorns in a food processer
or blender.

Melt the oil or butter in a frying pan, add the pepper
and stir. Fry for a couple of minutes. Add the leek and
fry for a couple of minutes. Pour over the cream and
add salt to taste. When it starts to thicken, add the
crème fraîche.

This sauce should be quite thick. A tablespoon of sauce
on each plate is usually enough, and it is quite hot.
Wonderful served with a good steak.

TIP
My teenagers enjoy this sauce, but
my youngest one finds it too strong.
For younger family members, mix
together 5 ml sauce with 30–45 ml
crème fraîche. This gives a milder
yet tasty sauce.

Mushroom sauce

4 servings

50 g organic coconut oil or butter
1 onion, chopped
100 g mushrooms, sliced (feel free to use a
   variety)
1–2 cloves garlic, crushed
Salt and pepper
30 ml Worcestershire sauce
200 ml fresh cream
200 ml crème fraîche

Melt the oil or butter in a frying pan and fry the onion for a couple of minutes. Add the mushrooms and fry for another couple of minutes. Add the garlic, seasoning and Worcestershire sauce. Pour in the cream and add the crème fraîche. Simmer for 5–8 minutes.

Remove from the heat and blend with a hand blender until smooth.

Serve with chicken or meat.

TIPS
- All kinds of mushrooms work with this sauce. Use your imagination or what's in season.
- If you prefer a thicker sauce, remove from the heat and stir in an egg yolk at the end. Alternatively, add 30–45 ml Philadelphia® cream cheese.

Heavenly sauce

4 servings

200 ml crème fraîche
200 ml fresh cream
15 ml Dijon mustard
15 ml tomato purée
5 ml paprika
Salt and white pepper
4 cloves garlic, crushed
15 ml dried tarragon

Mix all the ingredients together in a saucepan and bring to the boil. Reduce the heat and simmer for 7–9 minutes. If you prefer a runnier sauce, add more cream. If you want a thicker sauce, simmer for longer.

Serve with grilled chicken fillets or barbecued meat.

TIP
Always read the list of ingredients for the mustard you buy because it often contains lots of carbs. Dijon mustard is usually low in carbs.

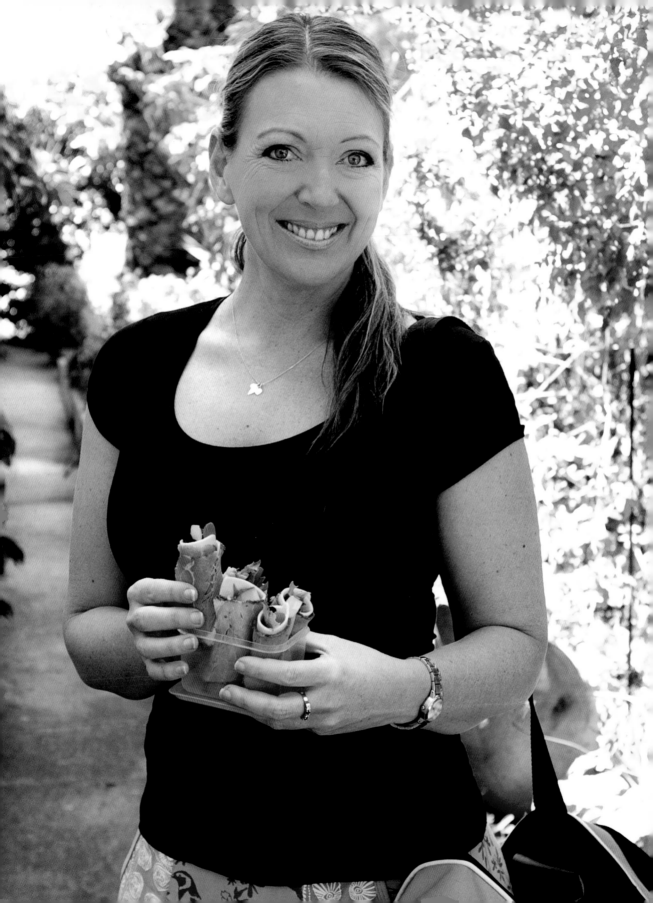

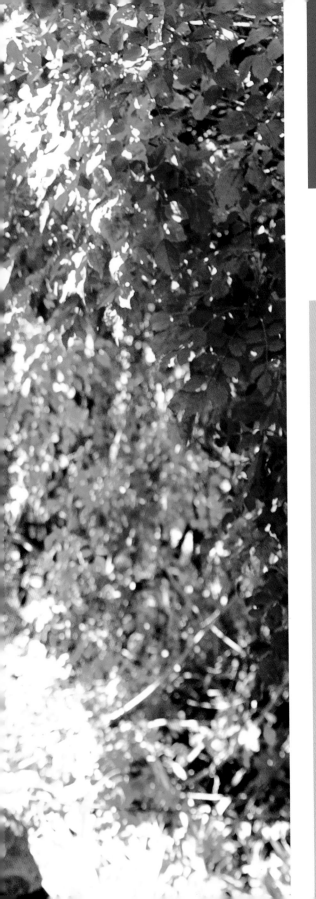

Healthy snacking

If you or the kids are hungry during the day, then a snack is a good choice - the right kind of snack.

The idea is not to snack all day long, but if there is a big gap between meals, or you are going to work out or the kids have sport activities, then a snack is probably a good idea.

The snacks given in this chapter are also good as after-training snacks and are a healthy alternative to tea-time snacks if you are having afternoon guests.

Snack time should not be used as an excuse to eat, so try to distinguish between being hungry and just feeling nibbly. Children use a lot more energy than adults, so they do tend to be hungrier more often and usually exhibit this need for food with a change in mood.

In this chapter the suggestions, tips, recipes and ideas for snacking will work for everyone, young and old. My snack ideas are quite similar to my breakfast suggestions, and can be easily interchanged.

Happy snacking!

Crisp bread sandwich

**2 pieces low-carb crisp bread per serving
(see page 37)**

Suggestions for sandwich fillings:

Butter, salami, Brie cheese and yellow pepper
Butter, ham, cheese and tomato
Butter, cheese and tomato
Butter, Brie cheese and avocado

All ingredients should be fresh and/or raw.

Cheese bombs
2–6 per serving

Use a cheese slicer and slice the cheese. Add 5 ml butter or Philadelphia® cream cheese, roll up and enjoy.

Cheese and salami rolls with peppers and apple
1 serving

4 slices cheese
4 slices salami or ham
20 ml butter or high-fat cream cheese
½ red, green or yellow pepper
**½ apple (for those who manage fruit in their diet
   – can be omitted)**

Layer the slices of cheese, salami or ham and 5 ml butter or cream cheese. Cut the pepper and apple into thin slices and place a slice of each on the cheese. Roll up. A good and healthy snack!

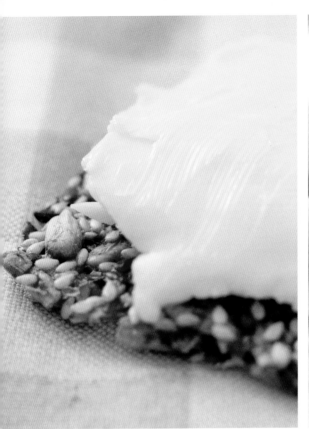
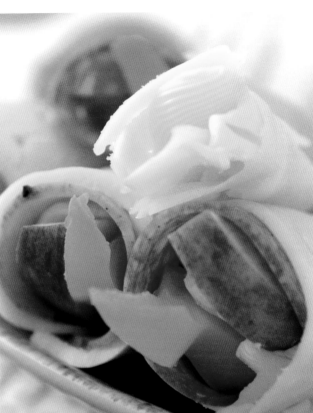
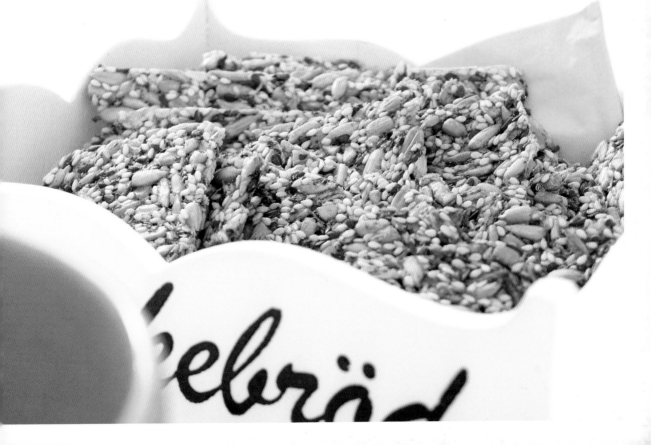

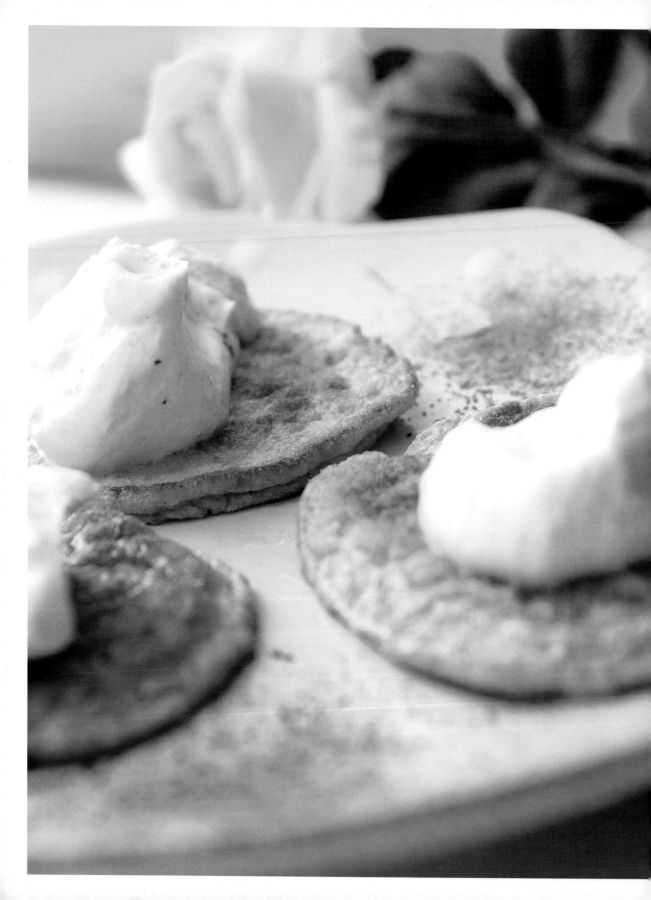

Pancakes

Makes 1 pancake

1 egg
15 ml psyllium husk (available from health
stores)
30 ml fresh cream
Seeds from ½ vanilla pod
15 ml organic coconut oil or butter

Serve with
100 ml whipped cream
100 ml fresh berries

Whisk the egg, psyllium husk, cream and vanilla together.

Melt the oil or butter in a frying pan. Pour the egg mixture into the pan and fry the pancake over low heat. Turn over when the underside is cooked. Cook the other side.

Serve with whipped cream and berries.

TIPS
- You can use apple instead of pear for the mini pancakes. You can also add 15 ml chopped nuts.
- This makes a lovely dessert, Sunday breakfast or a filling snack. My youngest daughter, who is not so fond of eggs, loves these pancakes.

Cinnamon and pear mini pancakes with vanilla cream

2 servings (4 mini pancakes)

1 small pear
1 egg
30 ml almond flour (available at health stores)
5 ml psyllium husk
5 ml ground cinnamon
15 ml butter
100 ml fresh cream
Seeds from ½ vanilla pod

Grate the pear with a cheese grater.

Whisk the egg and add the almond flour, psyllium husk and cinnamon. Add three-quarters of the pear and mix well.

Melt the butter in a frying pan and spoon tablespoonfuls of the pancake mixture into the pan to make four pancakes. Fry them for a few minutes, until set. Turn over and fry the other side.

Whip the cream and add the remainder of the grated pear and the vanilla.

Serve the pancakes with the cream.

VARIATION
If fruit is not part of your eating plan, you can use grated baby marrow instead. Squeeze out the water first and follow the recipe as above.

Easy-to-make children's smoothie

1 serving

100 ml fresh cream
100 ml Greek or Bulgarian yoghurt or plain yoghurt
100 ml frozen berries

Mix all the ingredients together in a blender. Serve immediately.

Apple and cinnamon smoothie

1 serving

15 ml butter
½ apple, peeled and chopped
5 ml ground cinnamon
100 ml fresh cream
100 ml Greek or Bulgarian yoghurt
Seeds from ½ vanilla pod
3–5 ice cubes

Melt the butter in a saucepan and add the apple chunks and the cinnamon. Simmer for 5–8 minutes until the apples are soft and mushy.

Mix all the ingredients, including the apple, together in a blender. Serve immediately.

Filling smoothie

2 servings

200 ml frozen berries
100 ml soda or sparkling water
200 ml fresh cream
1 avocado
1 egg yolk
Seeds from ½ vanilla pod
½ ripe pear (for children or those who do not need to restrict their fruit intake)

Mix all the ingredients together in a blender. Serve immediately.

Low-carb protein drink (egg milk) and hot chocolate

See page 41. Egg milk is great as a snack and really good just before or after a work-out.

TIPS

- Smoothies are great snacks for kids and adults, especially just before or after training.
- For adults, exchange the fruit for avocado to avoid fructose.
- Vanilla and cinnamon work well in most smoothies, as do nuts and egg yolk. This adds even more nourishment and makes you feel full.

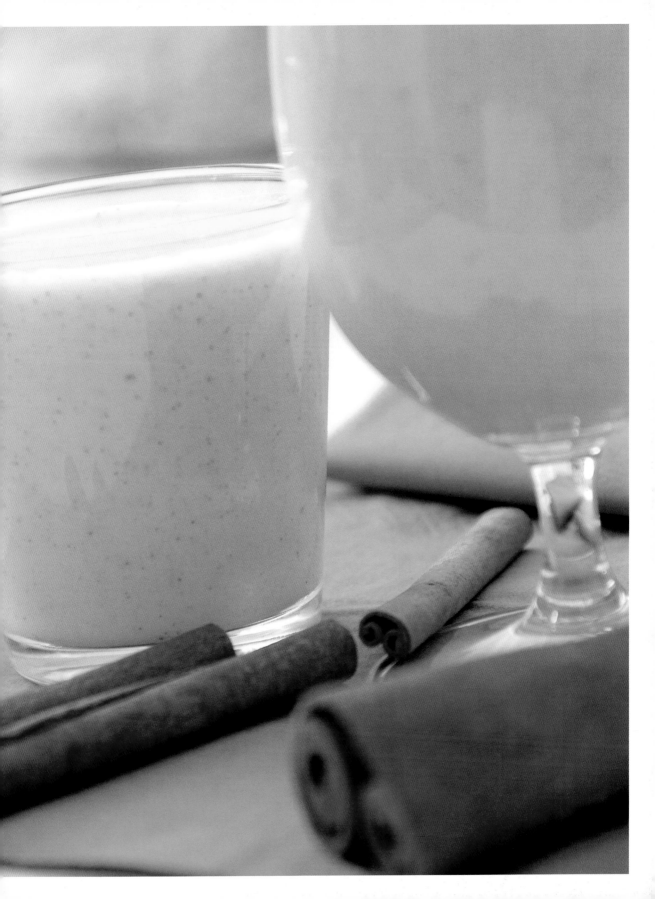

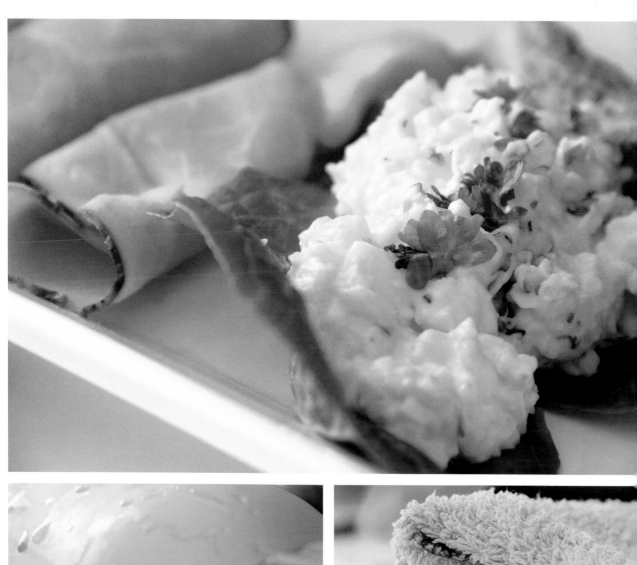

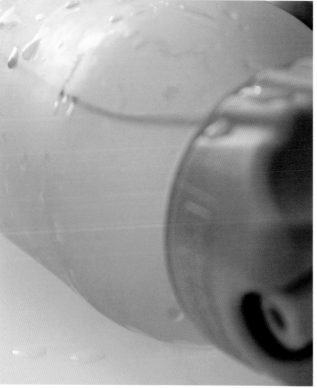

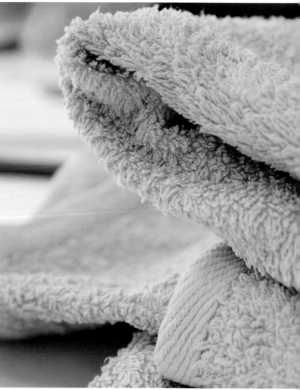

Egg snack
1 serving

1 hard-boiled egg
30 ml mayonnaise
5 ml butter
Salt and pepper
15 ml chopped fresh parsley

Mash the egg with a fork. Add the mayonnaise and the butter. Season with the salt, pepper and parsley.

Serve as is or on a lettuce leaf. Works well on slices of ham too.

TIP

If your child eats bread or the low-carb crisp bread on page 37, then this is lovely to have on top. It is quite filling too.

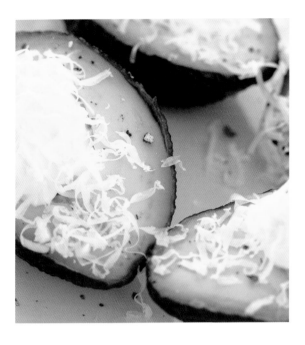

Avocado snack
2 servings

1 avocado, halved and depipped
Salt and pepper
30 ml mayonnaise
30 ml grated cheese

Season the avocado halves with salt and pepper. Spoon 15 ml mayonnaise on each half and sprinkle over the cheese.

TIPS

- An avocado contains 4.4 g carbs, 15.3 g fat and 2.0 g protein per 100 g. It also contains vitamin E (an antioxidant), magnesium, folic acid and potassium.
- Avocado has a wonderful consistency and is suitable for young children and babies.
- Avocados are easy to bring along in your bag or backpack as a snack.
- My children often have avocado as an accompaniment to dinner instead of potatoes, pasta or rice.

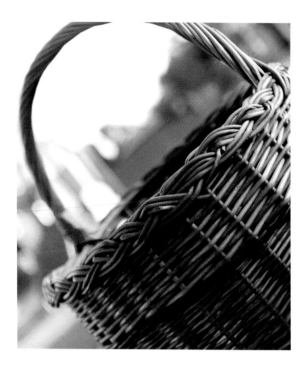

Apple snack with nut butter

2 servings

1 apple or pear, sliced
40 ml nut butter (macadamia nut butter, almond butter, peanut butter)

Slice the apple or pear and add 5 ml nut butter to each slice.

Picnic snacks

Sausages (at least 80% meat)
Egg wraps with favourite filling or with cheese and tomato (A wrap is an omelette (see page 34) consisting of 2 eggs and 30 ml fresh cream fried in butter. Leave to cool and then add a filling of your choice. Roll up to form a wrap.)
Cherry tomatoes
Avocado
Cubes of cooked chicken on a toothpick
Cheese cubes
Low-carb crisp bread (see page 37)
Nuts
Pepper rings (yellow, orange, red or green)
Rooibos tea in a thermos

Put together a mix of some of the above suggestions in different containers.

> **TIP**
> Nut butters are a great source of energy, but are also high in carbs, with peanut butter being the worst and macadamia nuts the best.

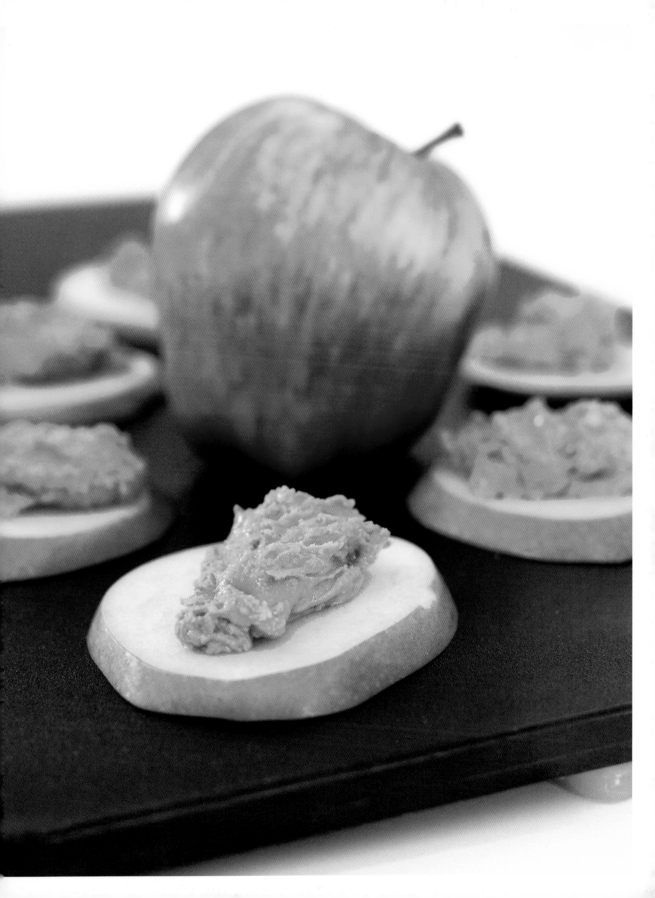

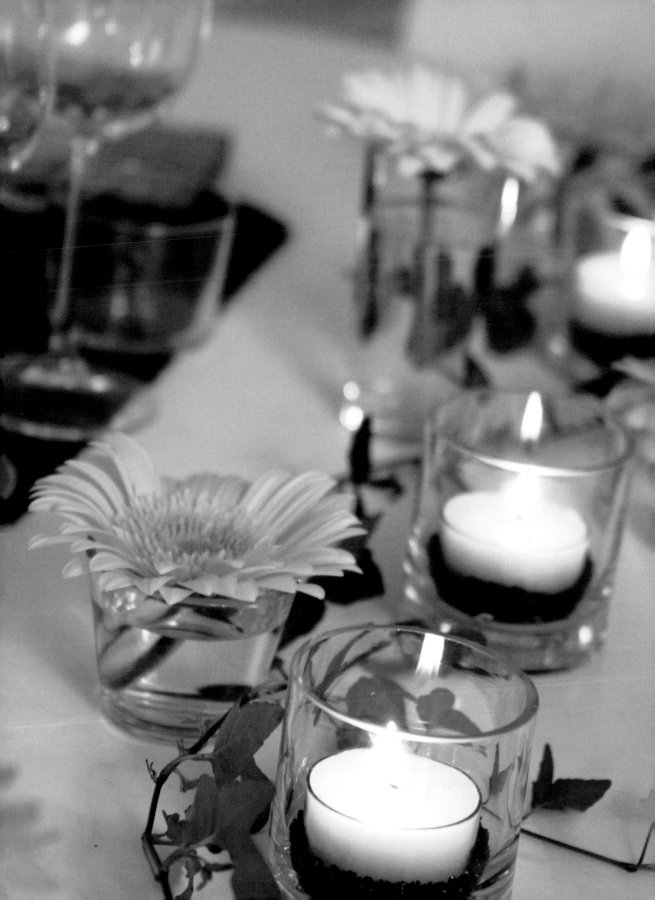

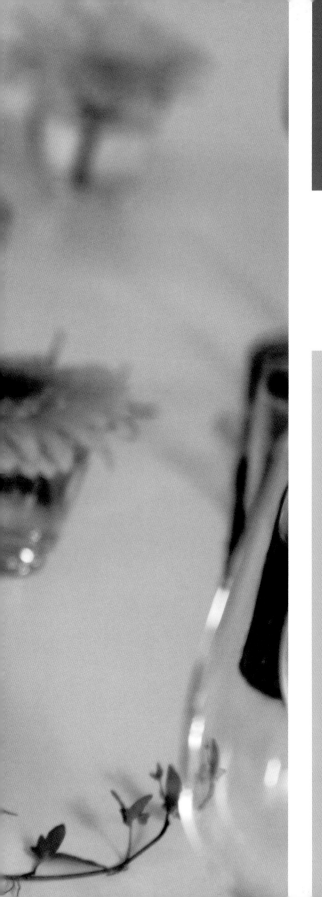

Desserts and festive moments

Celebrations, especially birthdays, and festive occasions such as Christmas, Easter, Valentine's day and Halloween are associated with sweet things.

Every now and then it's nice to enjoy a special treat after dinner or for afternoon tea, but sweet and sugar is not a must on these occasions. I will admit, however, that there aren't many LCHF sweets around that don't contain sugar or artificial sweetener.

I don't have any miracle solutions to this, as a low-carb cake without the sweet taste is not the same as the sweet version. If I do choose to make a dessert I always do it the LCHF way, without the sweetness, and I often serve some good cheese after a meal.

If I do bake or prepare a dessert, I use vanilla seeds, coconut or berries. For children I opt for homemade rather than bought sweets and cakes, and find that honey is a better choice of sweetener than sugar. I do, however, have a favourite that even my children enjoy, and that's my chocolate mousse.

Choose what suits you and your family. The level of sweetness will be determined by your needs and tolerance levels.

Monique's real chocolate mousse

6 servings

**200 g dark chocolate (at least 70% cocoa, but
    preferably above 80%)**
1 egg yolk
Pinch of salt
5 ml grated orange zest (optional)
50 ml organic coconut oil
500 ml fresh cream

Break the chocolate into pieces and melt in a bowl
suspended over simmering water.

Mix the egg, salt and orange zest together in a bowl.
If the coconut oil is solid, melt it so that it is in liquid
form. Slowly add the coconut oil to the egg mixture,
stirring all the time. Whip the cream lightly, not too stiff.

Add the oil and egg mixture to the melted chocolate
and stir together. Carefully fold the chocolate into the
whipped cream.

Pour the mousse into a large bowl or individual glasses
or bowls. Refrigerate for at least 1 hour. Remove from
the fridge 15 minutes prior to serving.

Decorate with cream and berries if you like.

TIPS

- If you are making the mousse for
  children, they will probably
  prefer the 70% cocoa chocolate.
- For those who are sensitive to
  sweet tastes, use the highest
  percentage cocoa chocolate that
  you can find. I use both 100%
  cocoa chocolate mixed with 85%
  or 90%.
- You can also make a berry purée to
  serve with the chocolate mousse.

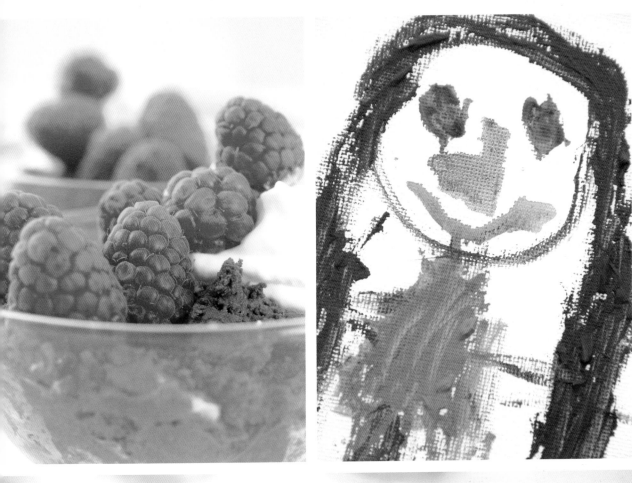
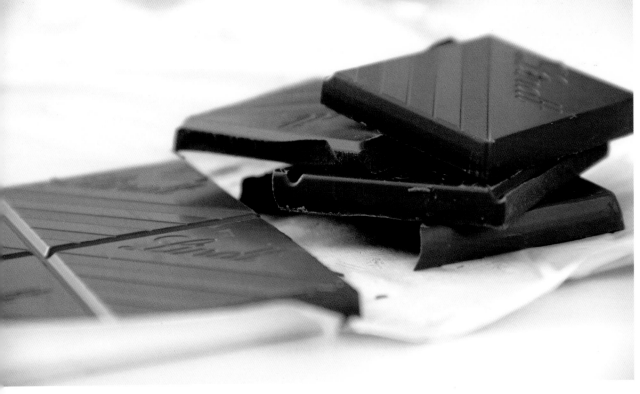

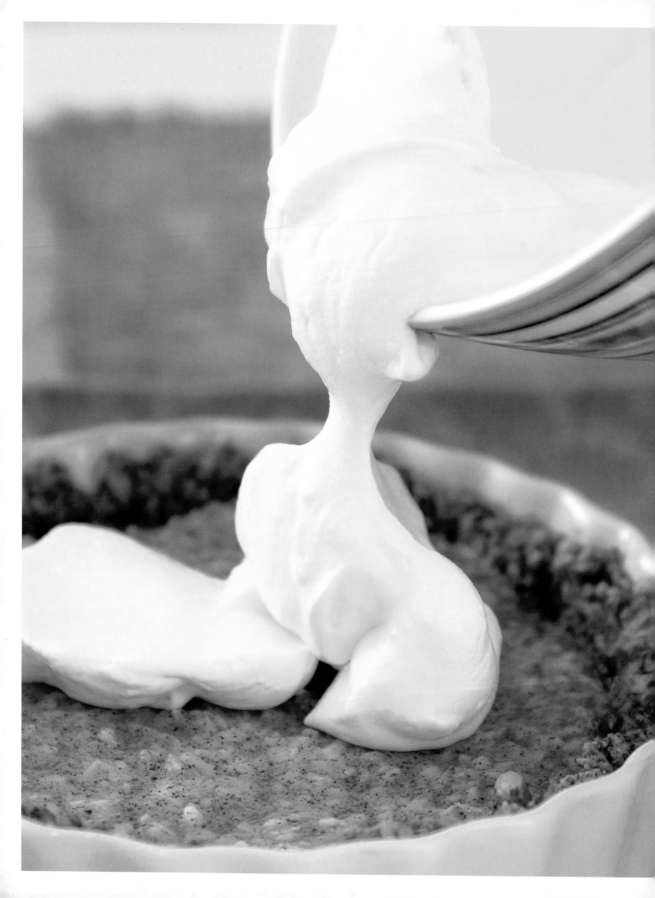

Low-carb cheesecake

Makes 1 cake (12 servings)

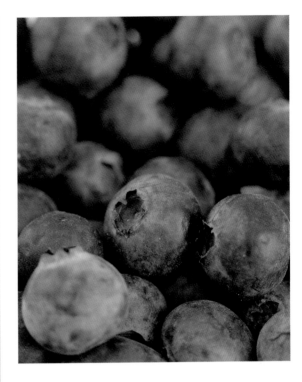

Crust

100 g butter
250 ml chopped mixed raw nuts
10 ml ground cinnamon
Seeds from ½ vanilla pod
200 ml desiccated coconut

Preheat the oven to 175 °C.

Melt the butter in a small saucepan. Mix all the remaining crust ingredients together and add the melted butter. Press the crust into a pie dish and bake for 5–10 minutes.

> **TIP**
> Make sure you use unsweetened vanilla if you choose to use vanilla essence as a substitute for vanilla pods.

Filling

300 g Philadelphia® cream cheese
2 eggs
Seeds from ½ vanilla pod
100 ml desiccated coconut

Using an electric beater, whip the cream cheese, eggs, vanilla and coconut together. Pour the filling onto the pie crust. Bake for 30 minutes and then remove from the oven and allow to cool.

Refrigerate until serving. (This is as far as you can prepare ahead of time.)

Topping

200 ml crème fraîche
Berries

Whip the crème fraîche with an electric beater and spread over the top of the baked cheesecake. Add the berries on top, in a heap.

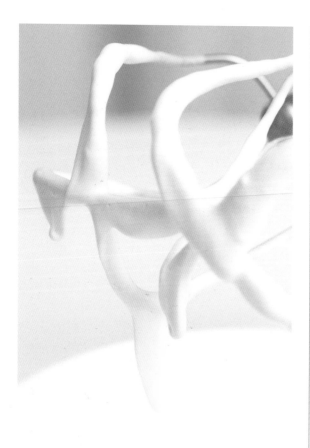

Raspberry (or other berry) mousse

4 servings

5 ml powder or 2 sheets gelatine
400 ml raspberries (or other berries)
Seeds from 1 vanilla pod
400 ml fresh cream

Prepare the gelatine according to the package instructions.

Place the berries in a saucepan and cook over medium to low heat for around 10 minutes. Blend until smooth using an electric hand mixer or food processor. Stir in the gelatine and vanilla while the berries are still warm. Set aside and allow to cool.

Whip the cream and then fold it into the cooled berry purée. Pour the mixture into small serving bowls, glasses or one large serving dish. Refrigerate for at least 2 hours.

Serve as is or with a spoon of whipped cream on top. You can also decorate with a small piece of dark chocolate.

TIP Blackcurrants make a great variation of this dessert.

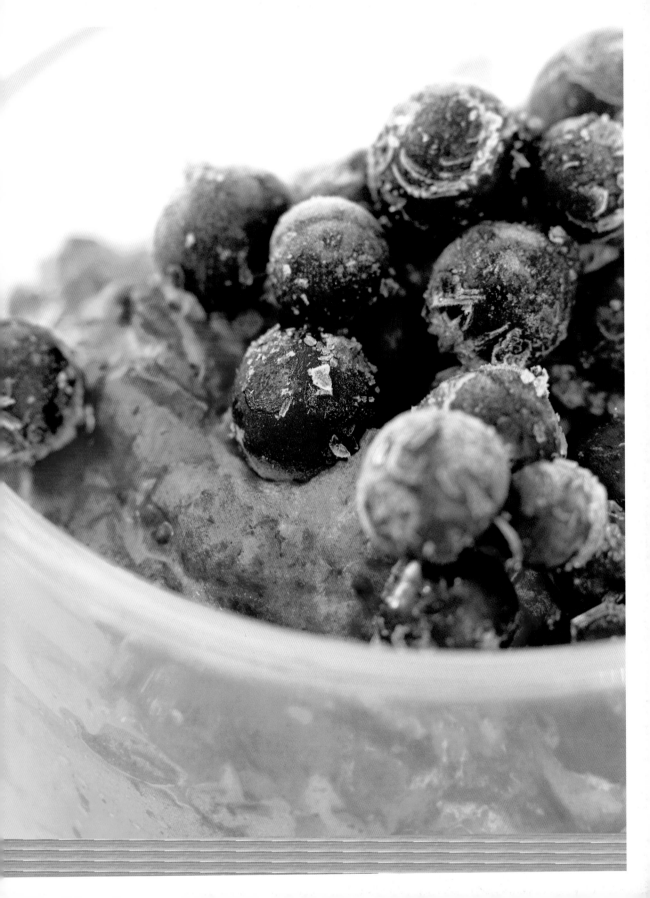

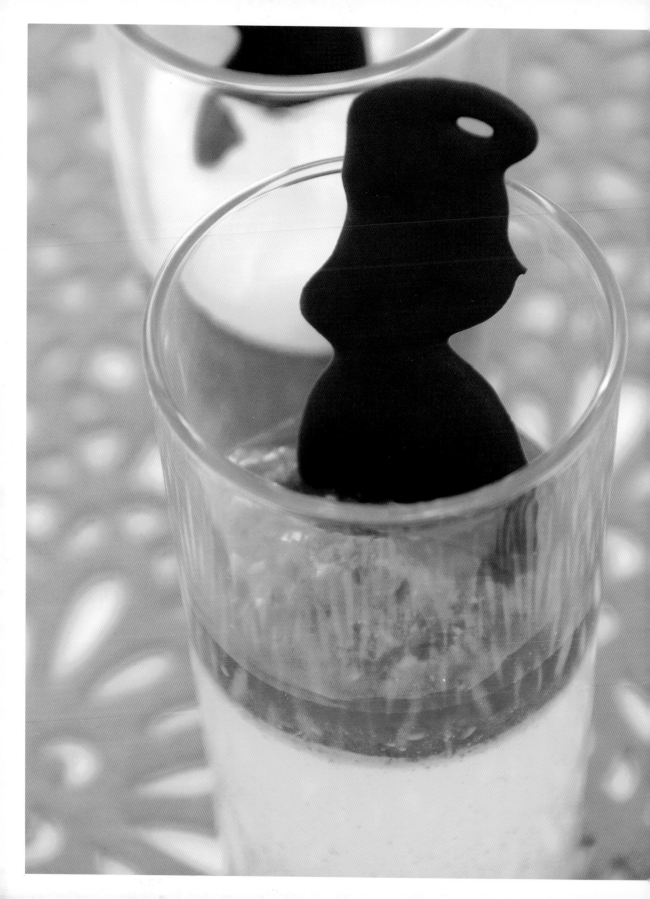

Panna cotta

6 servings

500 ml fresh cream
15 ml organic coconut oil
200 ml desiccated coconut
Seeds from 1 vanilla pod
5 ml powder or 2 sheets gelatine
Berries and/or coconut flakes for decorating

Pour the cream and coconut oil into a saucepan and bring to the boil. Add the desiccated coconut and the vanilla. Stir and remove from the heat.

Prepare the gelatine according to the package instructions. Add the gelatine to the mixture, stirring continuously.

Pour the panna cotta into small glasses or a large bowl. Refrigerate for at least 2 hours or until it's time to serve. Decorate with berries and/or coconut flakes.

VARIATION

To make chocolate panna cotta, grate 6 squares of dark (85% cocoa) chocolate and add it to the cream just before you pour the panna cotta into serving glasses. You can also melt the chocolate in the boiling cream for a smoother chocolate panna cotta.

TIP

Melt dark chocolate and get the kids to help make decorations for the dessert. Make sure you use greaseproof paper so that the chocolate does not stick to the work surface.

Pear and raspberry pie with a dash of lime cream

8 servings

30 ml butter
300 ml desiccated coconut
45 ml psyllium husk (available from health stores)
5 medium pears
200 ml chopped mixed raw nuts
100 ml sunflower seeds or pumpkin seeds
200 ml fresh cream
200 ml crème fraîche
Seeds from 1 vanilla pod
5 ml ground cardamom
100 ml raspberries

Preheat the oven to 180 °C. Grease a pie dish with the butter.

Sprinkle coconut onto the bottom of the prepared dish and sprinkle over the psyllium husk. Cut the pears into wedges or slices and place in the dish, covering the coconut. Sprinkle over the nuts and seeds.

Bring the cream, crème fraîche, vanilla and cardamom to the boil in a saucepan. Pour the cream mixture over the fruit in the pie dish and bake for 20–30 minutes.

Remove the dish from the oven and scatter the raspberries over the top of the pie. Return the pie to the oven and bake for another 7 minutes.

Lime cream
300–500 ml fresh cream
Grated zest of ½ lime

Whip the cream and add most of the lime zest. Save a pinch to sprinkle on top of the cream as garnish.

Serve the pie warm or cold with the lime cream.

TIP

I have a large pear tree at home, so I usually make this pie in the autumn when I have pears in the garden. You can use apples instead of pears and then add a touch of cinnamon, which is lovely with the apples.

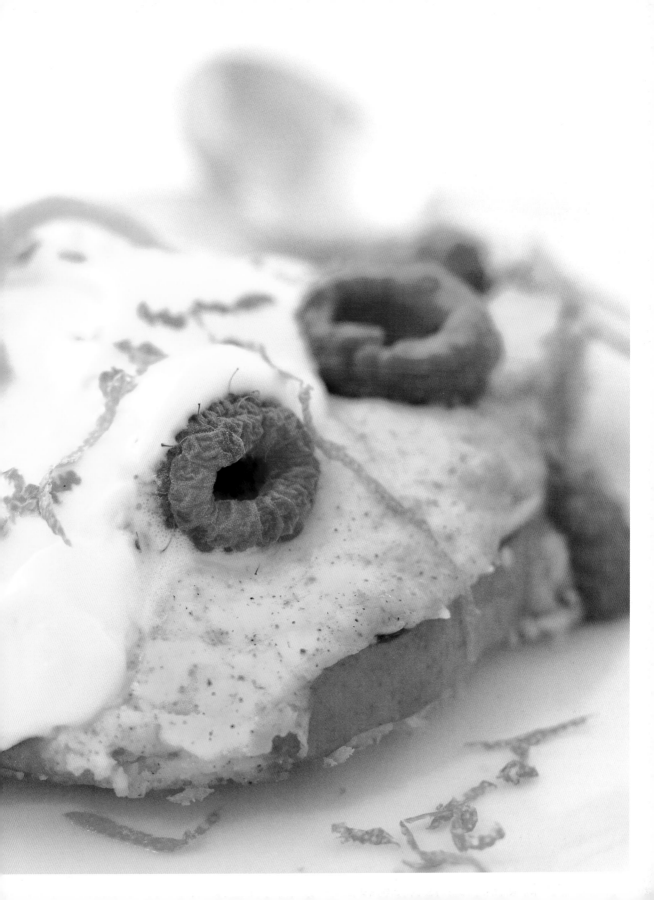

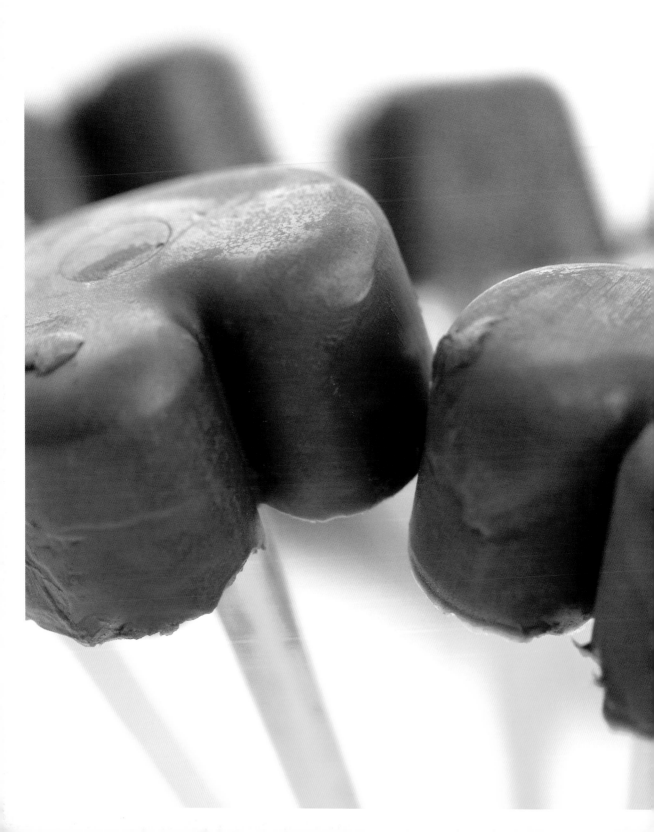

Chocolate lollipops

Makes 6

200 g dark chocolate (at least 70% cocoa, but preferably 90% cocoa)
1 red chilli, seeded and finely chopped (optional)
15 ml organic coconut oil

Set aside an ice cube tray.

Break up the chocolate and place in a bowl suspended over a pot of simmering water. Add the chilli and coconut oil to the melted chocolate.

Spoon the chocolate into each ice cube compartment. Place the tray in the fridge for a while until the chocolate starts to harden. Insert ice-cream or lollipop sticks before the chocolate hardens completely. Keep an eye on the chocolate so that the sticks don't fall over.

TIPS

- You can add whatever you like to the chocolate. Instead of chilli, try finely chopped nuts, desiccated coconut, vanilla seeds or goji berries.
- The chocolate lollipop is lovely to dip in a mug of hot coffee (for adults) or warm milk (for kids).
- The coconut oil may colour the chocolate white in places because the coconut oil turns white when cold.
- There are many different ice trays in various shapes that can be quite fun to use.

Cream cake

Makes 1 cake

Base

300 ml chopped almonds or mixed nuts
200 ml desiccated coconut
4 egg whites
Seeds from 1 vanilla pod

Preheat the oven to 150 °C. Draw three circles on baking paper, 18 cm in diameter. Place the baking paper on a baking tray.

Grind the nuts (fine or coarse) and mix with the coconut. Beat the egg whites until stiff and fold in the nut and coconut mixture and vanilla.

Spread the cake mixture within the circles on the baking paper and bake for 15 minutes. As soon as they are ready, loosen them from the paper. If they cool first, they will stick to the paper.

Filling

500 ml fresh cream
Berries, fruit or spice

Whip the cream until stiff. Choose one or two of the following fillings: clementine segments, mashed strawberries, pomegranate seeds, coarsely grated chocolate or cocoa powder, or cinnamon. (Or leave the cream plain.)

Place the first part of the cake base on a serving plate. Cover with whipped cream and whatever filling you decide to use. Place the next cake base on top of that and do the same with the cream and filling. Place the last cake layer on top and add cream. Decorate as you wish with grated dark chocolate or a few berries.

TIPS
- This cake works well for birthdays or afternoon tea.
- If you melt some dark chocolate in a bowl suspended over simmering water, you can blend that into the cream to make a chocolate cake. For kids, use a chocolate with a smaller percentage of cocoa if they don't like the darker chocolate.

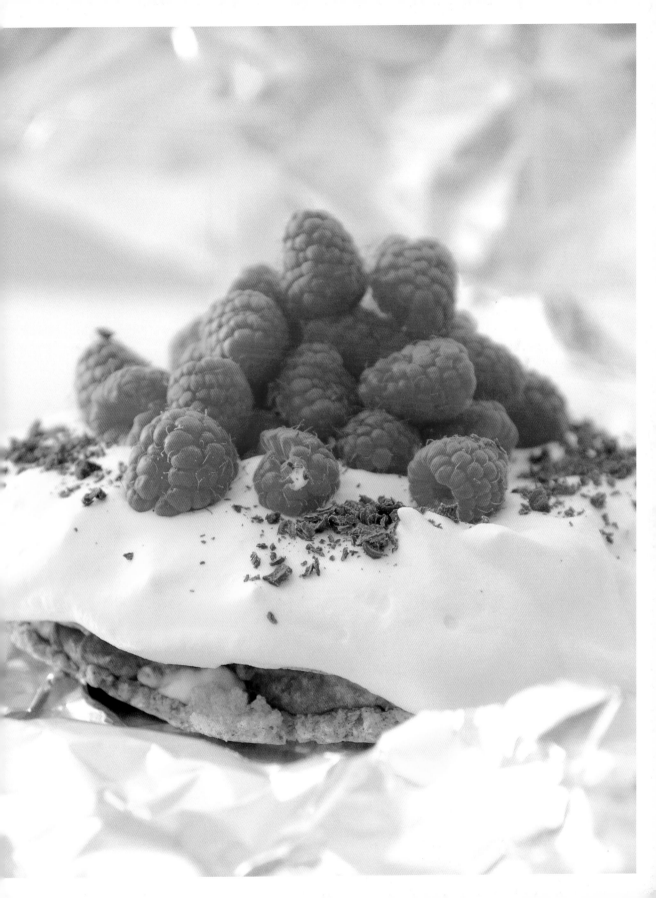

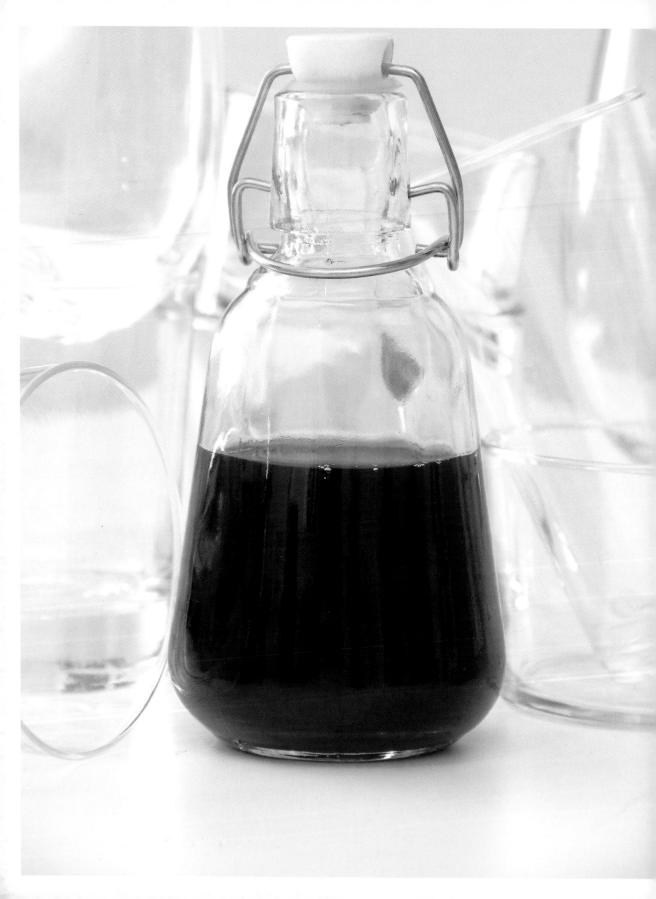

Low-carb cold drink/'juice' concentrate

Makes 1 litre

700 ml water
1 cinnamon stick
1 vanilla pod, split lengthways
Juice from 1 orange
300 ml mulberries (blackberries or strawberries can also be used)
300 ml raspberries
100 ml blueberries

Pour the water into a saucepan and add the cinnamon, the seeds from the vanilla pod and the orange juice. Add all the berries. Bring to the boil, then reduce the heat and simmer for 15 minutes. If it is very thick, add a little water. Remove the saucepan from the heat and leave to draw for 3 hours or overnight.

Strain the cold drink through a clean cloth or tea towel and pour into a bottle. Refrigerate. Add water to taste.

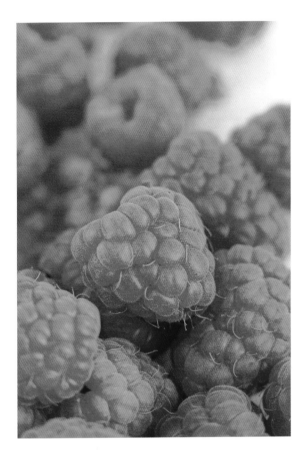

TIPS

- Use berries that are in season.
- To get a fizzy drink, you can mix the cold drink with sparkling water when serving.

Creamy pomegranate with pecan nuts

4 servings

500 ml fresh cream
1 pomegranate
200 ml pecan nuts, roughly chopped
2 squares dark chocolate, grated
Mint leaves for decorating

Whip the cream until quite stiff. Halve the pomegranate and hit the back with a big wooden spoon (or other large spoon) so that the seeds fall out. Mix the pomegranate seeds and nuts into the cream. Sprinkle the grated chocolate over the top and decorate with a mint leaf.

TIPS

- This dessert is very festive and perfect at Christmas time.
- You can exchange the pomegranate for clementine pieces or raspberries. You can even add vanilla seeds to get a slightly sweeter taste.

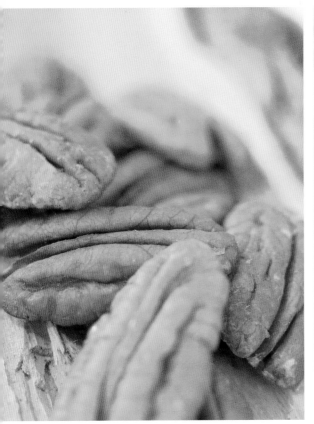
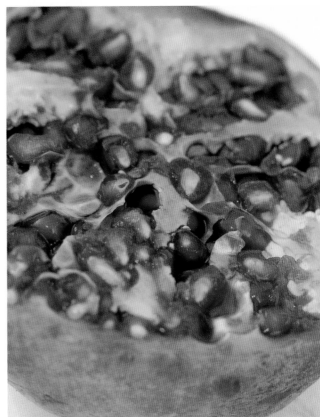
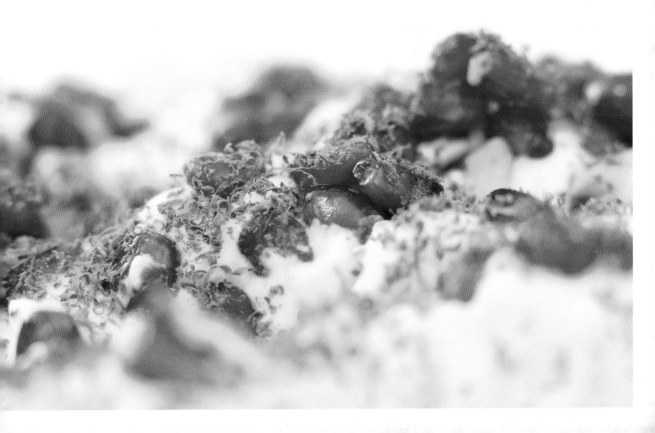

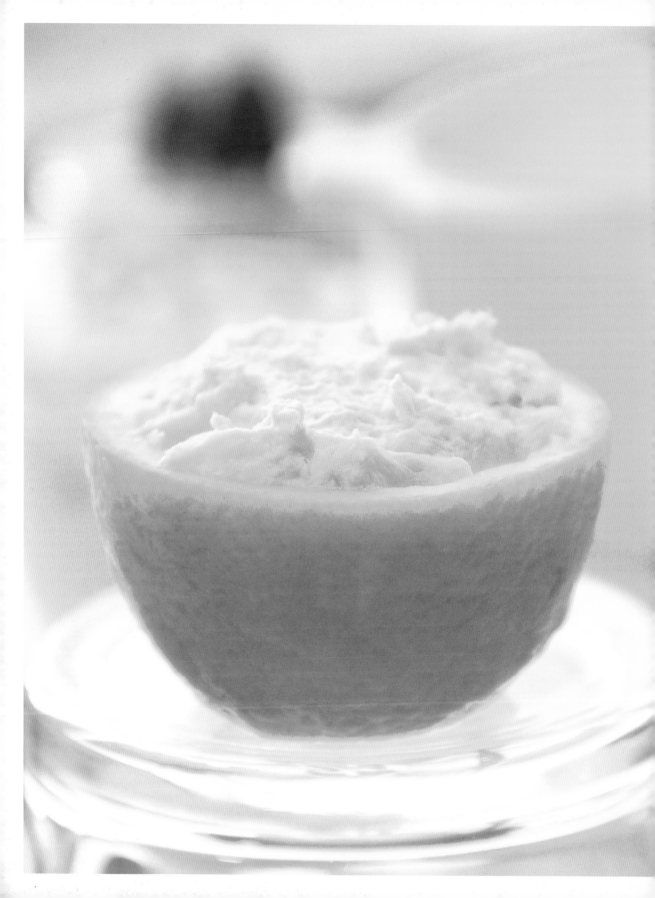

Low-carb ice cream

4–8 servings

Vanilla ice cream – basic recipe

300 ml fresh cream
Seeds from 1 vanilla pod
3 eggs, separated
250 g mascarpone cheese

Pour the cream into a bowl, add the seeds from the vanilla pod and whip the cream until thick. Whisk the egg yolks and add to the cream.

Stir the mascarpone until soft and add to the cream and egg mixture.

Whisk the egg whites until very stiff. Fold the egg whites gently into the cream mixture.

Pour the mixture into small cups or containers or a springform cake pan. If you use a springform pan, then line it with plastic wrap first so that you can easily remove the ice cream from the pan.

Freeze the ice cream for a minimum of 3 hours, but preferably overnight. Leave at room temperature for 10–20 minutes before serving.

TIPS

- Garnish the vanilla ice cream with berries, grated dark chocolate, grated lime or lemon zest, ground cinnamon or cocoa powder.
- You can also make ice lollies using ice-cream lolly moulds.

Strawberry ice cream

1 quantity vanilla ice cream (see left)
200 ml strawberries or other berries of your choice

Prepare the basic ice-cream recipe according to directions. Blend the berries with an electric hand blender or food processor and stir the berry purée into the vanilla ice cream. Freeze as instructed.

Chocolate ice cream

1 quantity vanilla ice cream (see left)
150 g dark chocolate (at least 70% cocoa)

Prepare the basic ice-cream recipe according to directions. Melt the chocolate in a bowl suspended over a saucepan of simmering water. Remove from the heat and leave to cool for a short while. Fold the chocolate into the vanilla ice cream. Freeze as instructed.

Lemon ice cream

1 quantity vanilla ice cream (see left)
2 lemons

Prepare the basic ice-cream recipe according to directions. Halve the lemons and squeeze out the juice. Clean out the lemons so that all the lemon flesh has been removed from the lemon halves. Mix the lemon juice with the vanilla ice cream and freeze as instructed.

To serve, cut off a small piece of the base of each lemon half so that they stand upright. Fill the lemon halves with the ice cream.

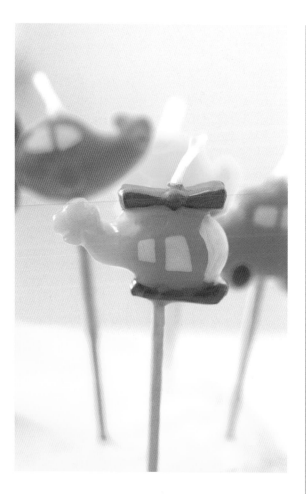

You can also freeze the ice cream in a bowl. Before serving, remove the bowl from the freezer and leave out for 10-15 minutes to allow it to soften slightly. Using a spoon, scoop out chunks of ice cream and place in individual bowls. Whip the cream and pipe it on top of the bowl of ice cream. Halve the berries and arrange them on top. This is perfect for children's birthday parties.

TIP

Ice-cream cake

8 servings

1 quantity vanilla ice cream (see page 171)
300 ml fresh cream
500 ml strawberries or raspberries (save a few for decorating)

Line a springform cake pan with plastic wrap. Pour the ice-cream mixture into the pan and freeze for at least 3 hours, but preferably overnight.

Remove from the freezer and place the ice cream on a large serving platter. Do this 15 minutes before covering and decorating the cake with the cream.

Whip the cream and purée the berries. Cover the cake with the berry purée and then cover the whole cake with whipped cream. Decorate with a few of the reserved berries. Serve immediately.

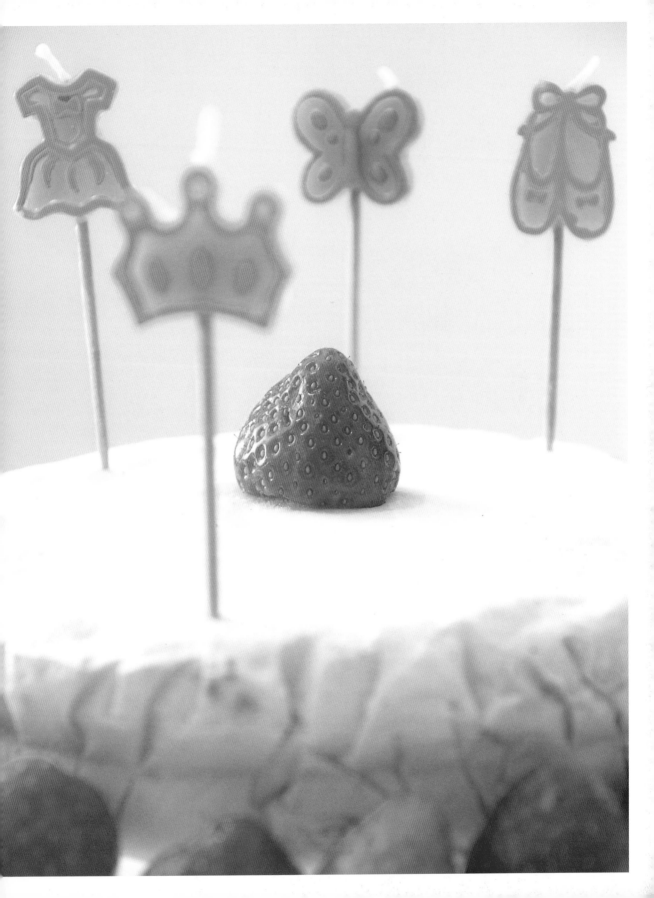

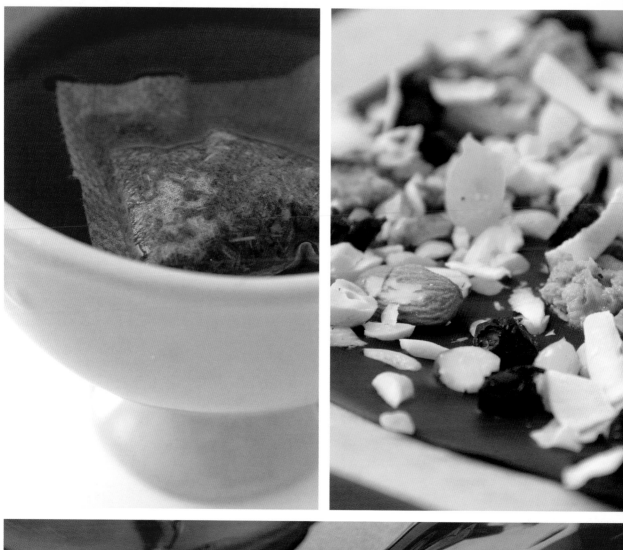

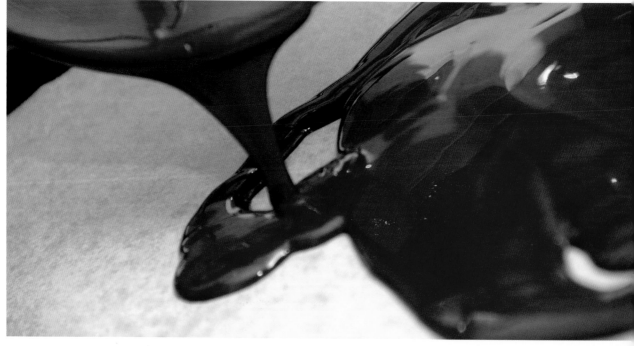

Low-carb treats

100 ml blueberries
200 g dark chocolate (85–90% cocoa)
Seeds from 1 vanilla pod
5 ml grated orange zest
30 ml pistachio nuts, coarsely chopped
30 ml cashew nuts, coarsely chopped
15 ml peanuts, coarsely chopped
30 ml pine nuts, coarsely chopped
15 ml desiccated coconut
30–45 ml macadamia nut butter (or unsweetened peanut butter)
1 dried apricot, finely chopped (optional)

Preheat the oven to 180 °C.

Place the blueberries on a baking tray lined with baking paper and 'dry' them in the oven for 45 minutes.

Melt the chocolate in a bowl suspended over simmering water. Remove from the heat and add the vanilla and orange zest.

Pour the chocolate onto greaseproof paper and sprinkle with the nuts and coconut. Using a teaspoon, distribute the nut butter evenly all over the chocolate and nuts, in small heaps. Distribute the berries over the top.

Sprinkle the apricot pieces on top. Refrigerate until the chocolate hardens. Break into smaller pieces before serving and place in a serving bowl or on a plate.

TIPS
- This is a wonderful treat at Christmas time or for parties.
- Have a piece with a cup of coffee after dinner, just not too often!
- Make sure you use unsweetened vanilla if you choose to use vanilla essence as a substitute for vanilla pods.

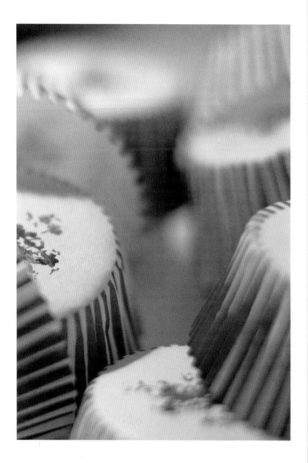

Lemon coconut tops

Makes 15–20

50 g butter
200 g desiccated coconut
2 eggs
Seeds from 1 vanilla pod
Grated zest and juice of ½ lemon
100 g dark chocolate (at least 70% cocoa, but
preferably 90%) (optional)

Preheat the oven to 175 °C. Line a baking tray with baking paper.

Melt the butter in a saucepan and add the coconut. Remove from the heat and stir in the eggs and vanilla. Add the lemon zest and juice and mix well.

Shape the mixture, using your hands, into small tops and place on the prepared baking tray. Bake for 15–20 minutes. Allow to cool.

Melt the chocolate in a bowl suspended over a saucepan of simmering water. Dip the bottom of each coconut top in the chocolate and place on greaseproof paper until the chocolate hardens. Place each coconut top in a mini cupcake cup.

TIP

You can also use this recipe for a cake base. Draw circles on baking paper and spread the coconut mixture in the circle. Bake in the oven until golden in colour. Add whipped cream and/or berries on top.

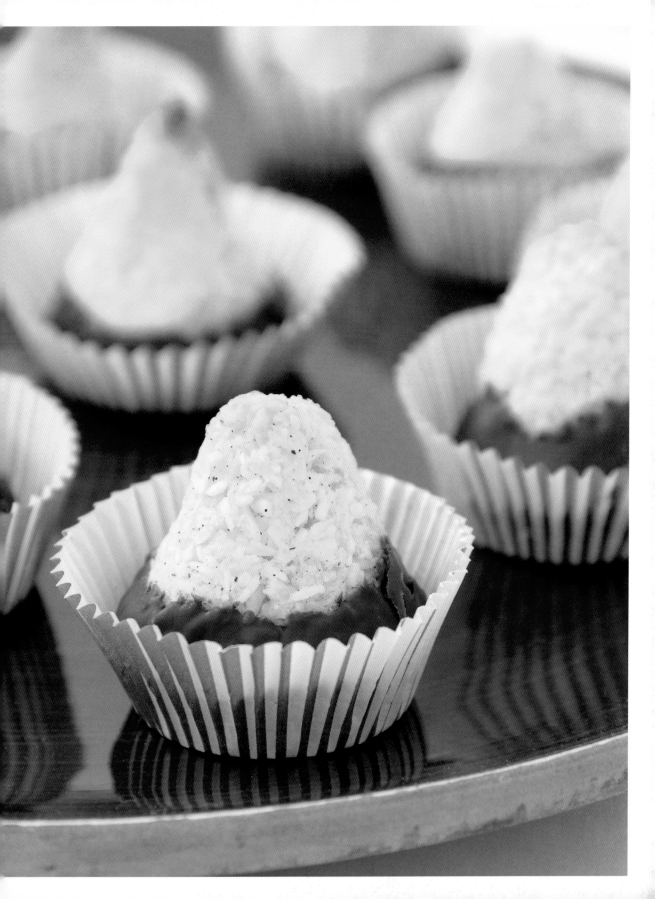

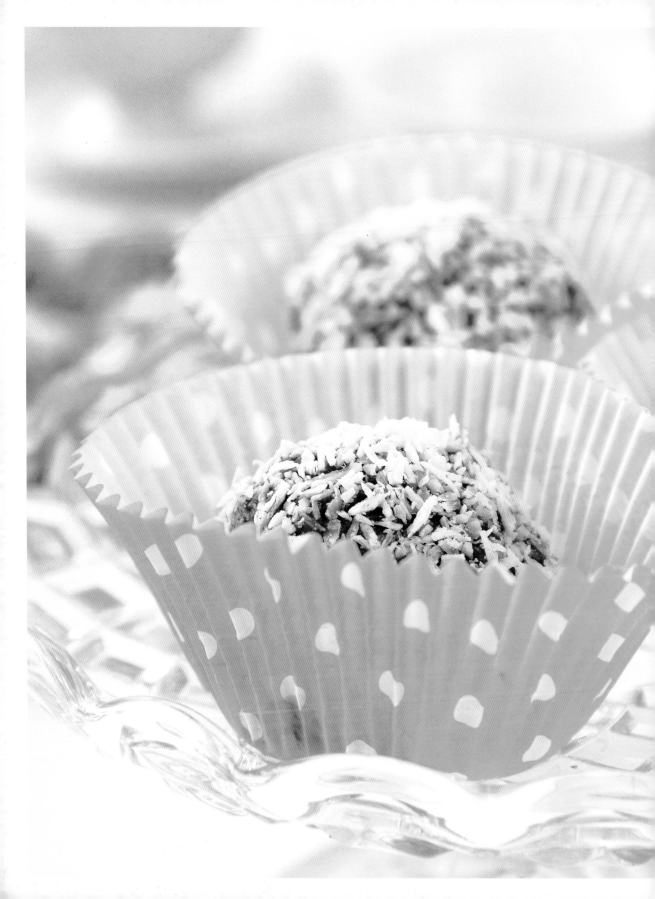

Chocolate balls

100 ml coconut cream
75 g butter
75 g organic coconut oil
100 ml raw mixed nuts, finely chopped (optional)
100 ml desiccated coconut
2 egg yolks
30 ml cocoa powder
Seeds from 1 vanilla pod
extra chopped nuts or desiccated coconut for
    coating

Separate the thick creamy part of the coconut cream
from the liquid (it's usually in a lump). Only use the
thick cream. Add the rest of the ingredients and mix
well. Using your hands, roll the mixture into balls, any
size you like.

Roll the balls in some chopped nuts or desiccated
coconut.

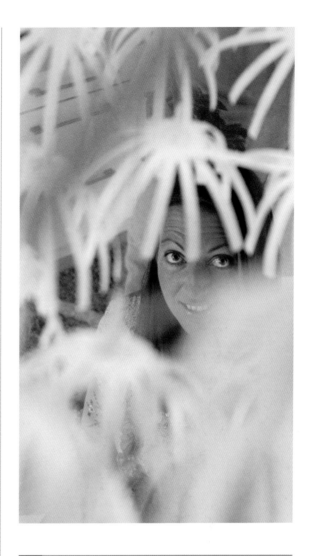

TIPS

⟋ Coconut oil becomes liquid at 24 °C,
so if the oil is in the fridge or in a
cool cupboard you may need to warm
it slightly in order to make it more
manageable.
⟋ If the chocolate mixture is too
runny, refrigerate it for a while to
harden slightly and make it easier
to roll into balls.

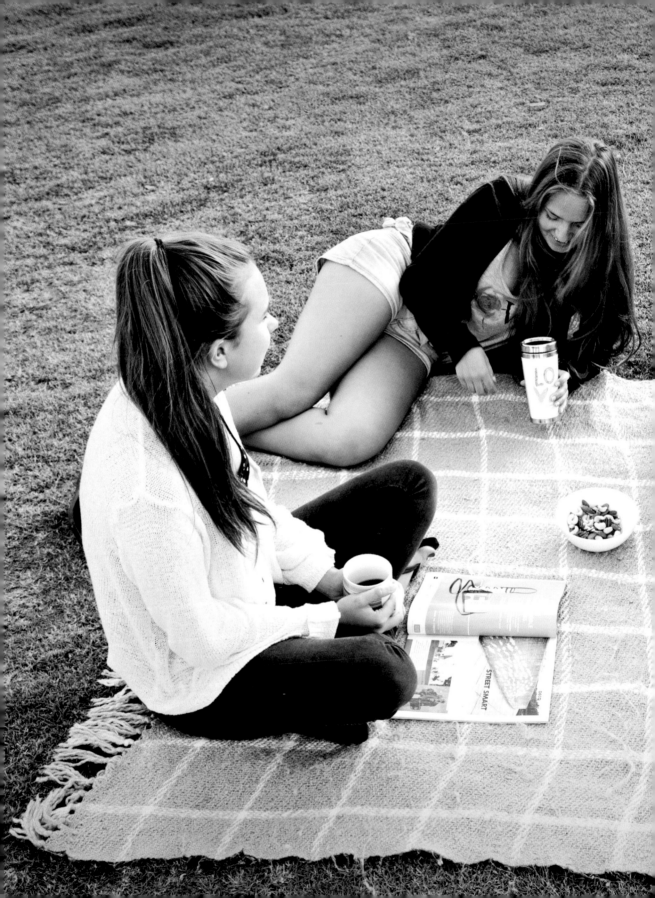

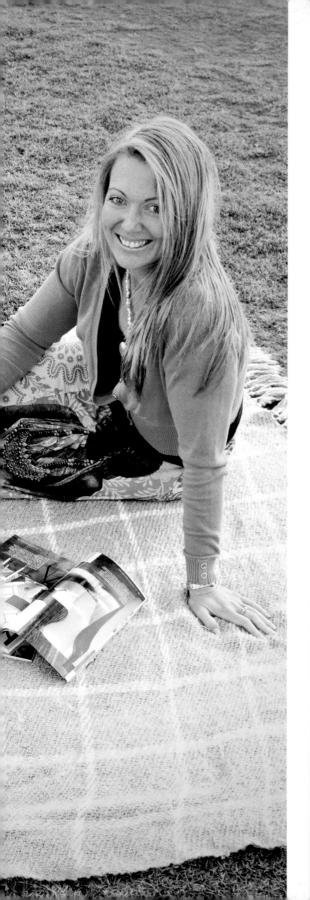

Weekend snacks

Weekends are often associated with time spent with family and friends, whether it's a get-together on a Friday evening, a family moment in the park or a festive dinner with friends, and much of this time involves food.

We also tend to eat more on weekends and different compared to the rest of the week – think party foods, fast foods, candy, chips, sodas or picnics.

In my family we have a tradition that Saturday is 'candy day'. It is the only day in the week that the kids are allowed to eat a bit of candy – but one day a week is enough. I try to associate the weekend with family and friends and good food, so instead of chips, candy and soda I make my own snacks for the family.

There are very good low-carb alternatives to make and eat on weekends. In this chapter I give you some ideas for healthy alternatives for weekend snacking or snacking in general.

I don't give servings for snacks because the LCHF method means you generally eat until you are full and this depends on the individual and how hungry you are.

Cheese chips

Use a good Cheddar cheese or another hard, tasty cheese.

Preheat the oven to 200 °C.

Slice the cheese with a cheese slicer, fold double and arrange on a baking sheet or tray. Leave some space between the slices so that they don't all melt together.

Place the tray on the top shelf of the oven for 3–6 minutes. Keep an eye on the cheese because once it starts to colour, it can burn very quickly. You want it to become crisp.

You can also prepare these chips in the microwave. Prepare in the same way and place the cheese on baking paper in the microwave. Microwave at 100% power for 3–5 minutes, watching that the cheese doesn't burn.

As soon as the cheese chips are ready, remove from the heat and place on a plate to cool.

Serve as is or with soup or some butter on each chip.

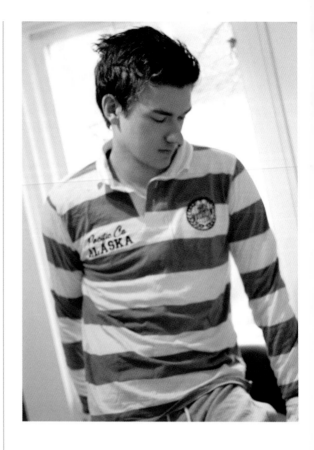

TIP

Spice the cheese chips with salt and/or pepper, chilli powder or any other favourite spice.

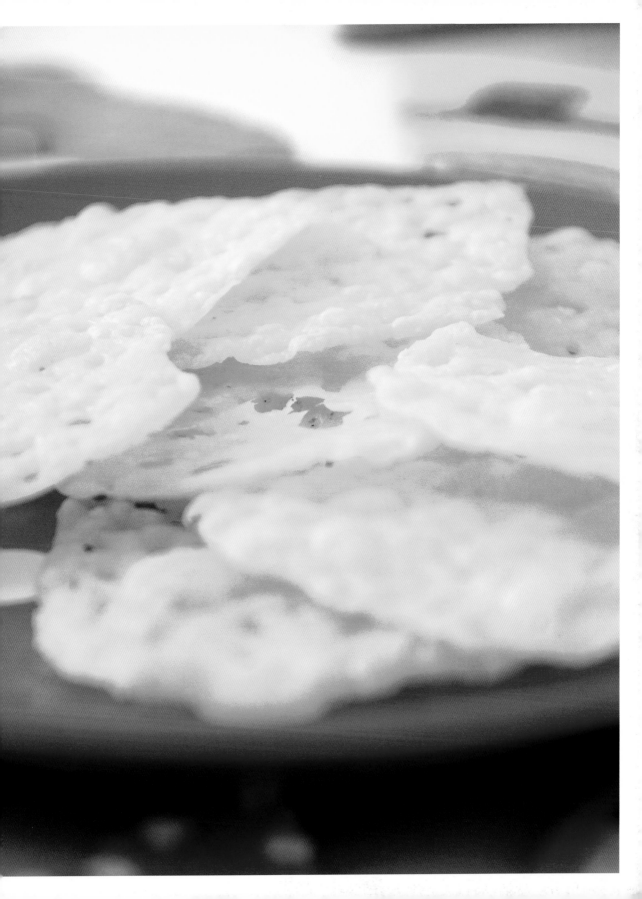

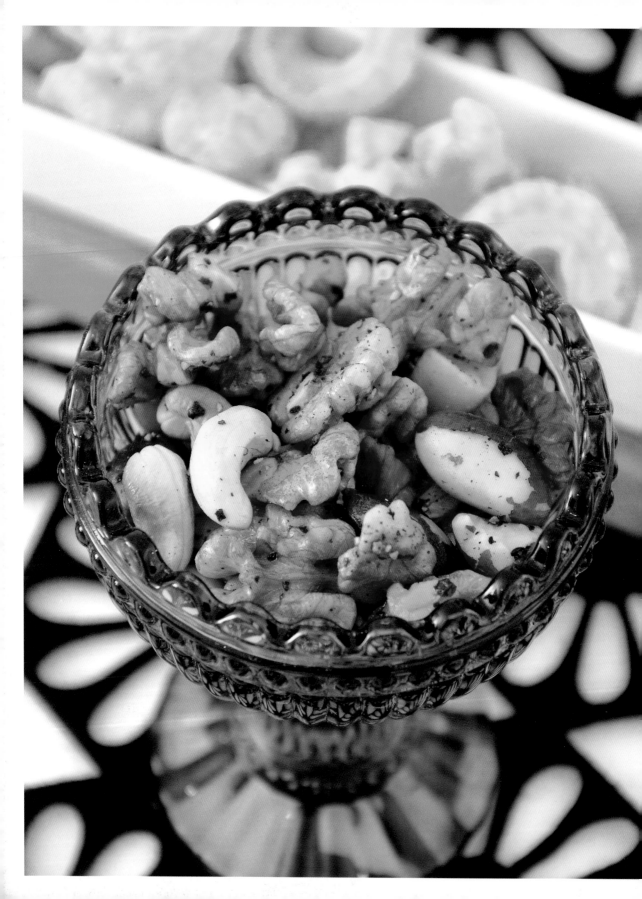

Pepper nuts

100 ml raw nuts of choice
5 ml olive oil
5 ml freshly ground black pepper

Place the nuts in a small freezer bag and add the oil and pepper. Hold the bag closed and shake it well so that the nuts are coated with the oil and pepper.

Heat a frying pan and fry the nut mixture for a few minutes, shaking the pan every now and then. Place in a serving bowl and enjoy.

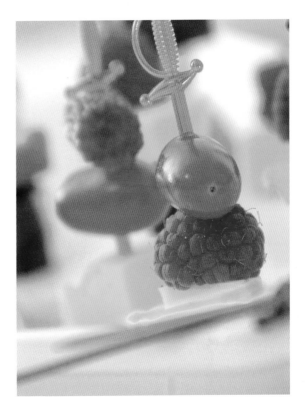

Party skewers

Use any skewers you have to hand.

Cocktail tomatoes
Peppers
Cheese
Raspberries
Cooked sausages (at least 80% meat)

Cut up the ingredients into bite-sized pieces and allow three to four pieces per skewer.

TIP Use any of your favourite vegetables, homemade meatballs or olives. Use ingredients that you and your kids enjoy.

Cheese and nut balls

200 g blue cheese
200 g Philadelphia® cream cheese
100 ml chopped raw nuts of choice

Mash the two cheeses together and roll into bite-sized balls. Roll the cheese balls in the chopped nuts.

Herb and cheese balls

200 g goat's cheese
200 g Philadelphia® cream cheese
100 ml finely chopped fresh dill (or any other favourite herb)

Mash the two cheeses together and roll into bite-sized balls. Roll the cheese balls in the chopped dill.

> **TIP**
>
> You can use just about any favourite spice or herb to coat the cheese balls. Cinnamon is very nice, as is chopped salted peanuts (if you eat those) or finely chopped chilli. Chopped goji berries can add a bit of sweetness.

Pear snacks with cheese

1 pear, cut into 8 slices
8 slices cheese
8 walnuts

Preheat the oven to 180 °C.

Place the pear slices on a baking sheet or tray. Lay 1 slice of cheese on each slice of pear. Place a walnut in the centre of each pear snack.

Grill the cheese in the oven for 15 minutes, or until the cheese has a golden brown colour.

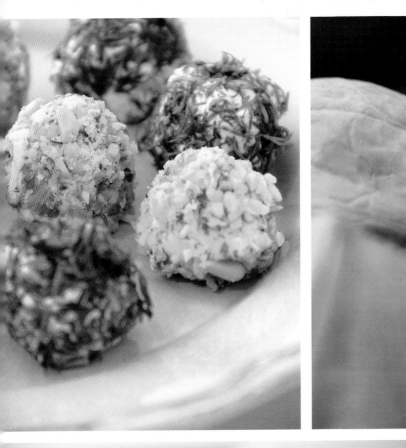

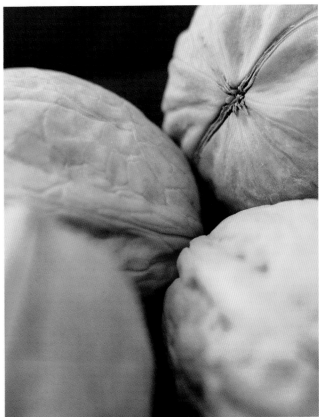

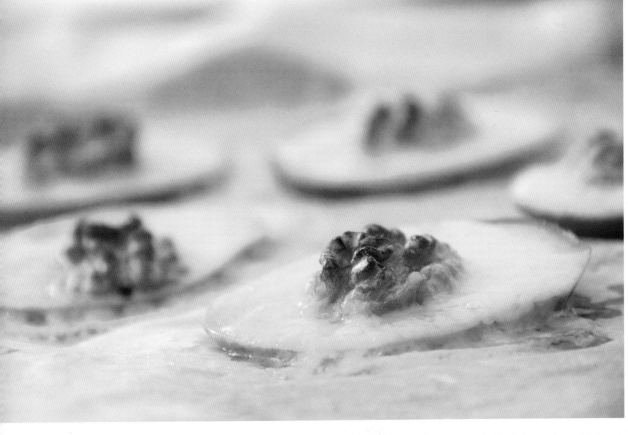

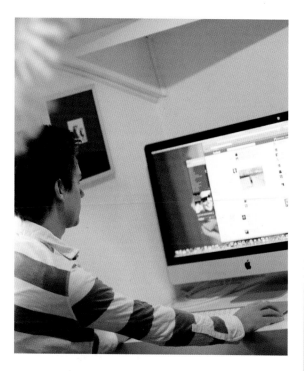

TIP

If you want a sweeter version, use chopped dried apricots or goji berries. Although not really recommended, the kids usually prefer this one and I'd say it's a better choice than any bought candy or chocolate bars!

Chocolate and nut bars

300 g dark chocolate (70–90% cocoa)
200 g sugar-free peanut butter
Pinch of salt
100 ml chopped raw nuts of choice
100 ml chopped salted peanuts

Line the bottom of a springform cake pan with baking paper.

Melt 150 g chocolate in a bowl suspended over a saucepan of simmering water. Pour the melted chocolate into the prepared pan and leave to cool for a short while. Spread the peanut butter over the chocolate and spread out all the chopped nuts on top of that. Sprinkle with the salt.

Melt the rest of the chocolate and pour it over the nuts so that they are completely covered. Place in the fridge and let it set for a couple of hours.

Cut into pieces around 3 x 3 cm in size. Serve straight away as they melt quite quickly, otherwise store in the fridge until needed.

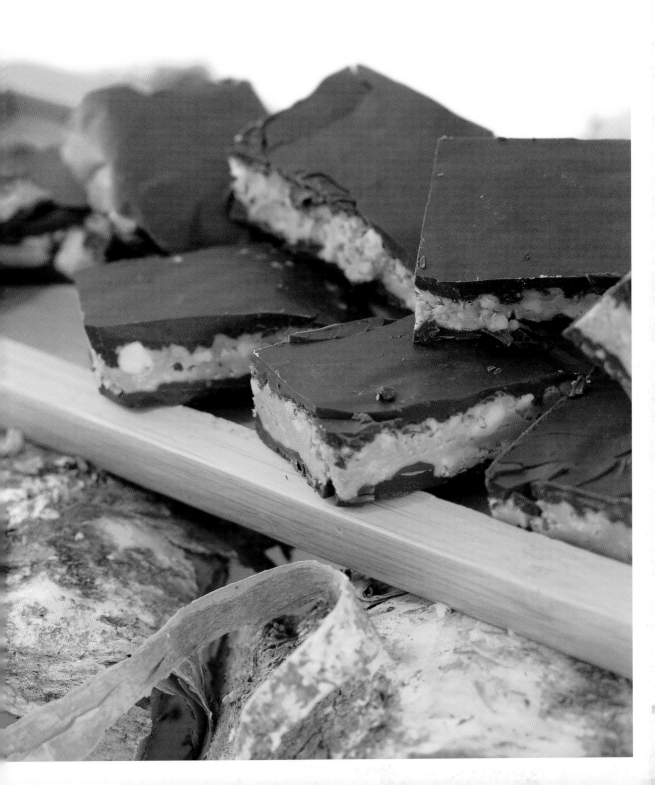

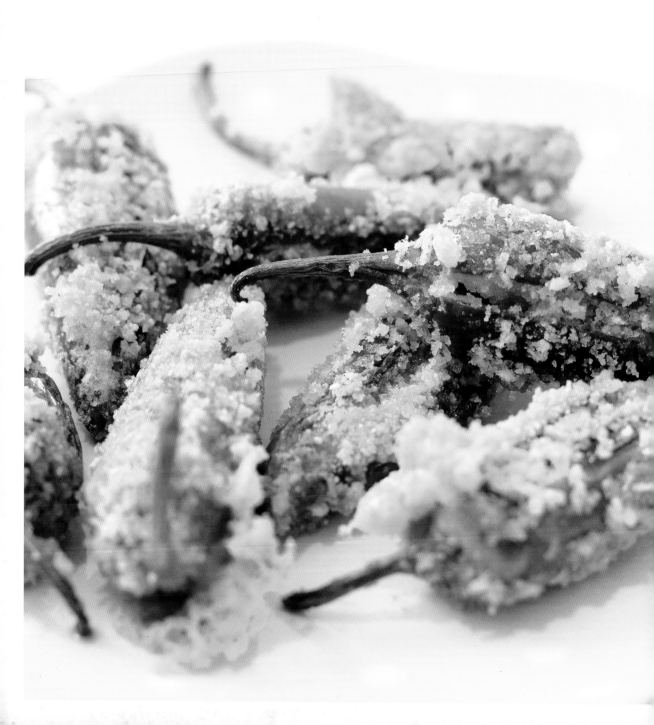

Chilli and cheese poppers

8 jalapeño chillies
Cheddar cheese
150 g pork rind snacks
1 egg, beaten
75 g organic coconut oil

Make a small incision along the side of each jalapeño and remove all the seeds from inside. Grate the Cheddar cheese or cut into pieces and fill each jalapeño with cheese. Close up.

Process the pork rinds until they form a powder (which you use instead of flour). Dip each jalapeño in the beaten egg and then cover with the pork rind 'flour'.

Heat the coconut oil in a frying pan and fry the jalapeño poppers until they have a lovely golden colour.

TIPS
- This recipe also works well with cream cheese or mozzarella.
- Jalapeños are not recommended for children. Use mozzarella cheese and make mozzarella sticks in the same way.

Recipe index